P9-CQW-221

PC
5?
.G53
2010

ALCOHOLISM

ALCOHOLISM

Maria Gifford
With
Stacy Friedman and Rich Majerus

Biographies of Disease

Julie K. Silver, M.D., Series Editor

GREENWOOD PRESS
An Imprint of ABC-CLIO, LLC

A B C 🞄 C L I O

Santa Barbara, California • Denver, Colorado • Oxford, England

Copyright © 2010 by Maria Gifford

All rights reserved. No part of this publication may be
reproduced, stored in a retrieval system, or transmitted,
in any form or by any means, electronic, mechanical,
photocopying, recording, or otherwise, except for the
inclusion of brief quotations in a review, without prior
permission in writing from the publisher.

Library of Congress Cataloging-in-Publication Data
Gifford, Maria.
    Alcoholism / Maria Gifford ; with the assistance of
Stacy Friedman and Rich Majerus.
        p. cm. — (Biographies of disease)
    Includes bibliographical references and index.
    ISBN 978-0-313-35908-8 (hard copy : alk. paper) —
ISBN 978-0-313-35909-5 (ebook)
    1. Alcoholism—Popular works. I. Title.
    RC565.G53 2010
    616.86'1—dc22   2009035274

14 13 12 11 10   1 2 3 4 5

This book is also available on the World Wide Web as an eBook.
Visit www.abc-clio.com for details.

ABC-CLIO, LLC
130 Cremona Drive, P.O. Box 1911
Santa Barbara, California 93116-1911

This book is printed on acid-free paper ∞
Manufactured in the United States of America

45.53

To Karl, in hopes of escaping it

Contents

Series Foreword

Every disease has a story to tell: about how it started long ago and began to disable or even take the lives of its innocent victims, about the way it hurts us, and about how we are trying to stop it.

In this Biographies of Disease series, the authors tell the stories of the diseases that we have come to know and dread. The stories of these diseases have all of the components that make for great literature. There is incredible drama played out in real-life scenes from the past, present, and future. You'll read about how men and women of science stumbled trying to save the lives of those they aimed to protect. Turn the pages and you'll also learn about the amazing success of those who fought for health and won, often saving thousands of lives in the process.

If you don't want to be a health professional or research scientist now, when you finish this book you may think differently. The men and women in this book are heroes who often risked their own lives to save or improve ours. This is the biography of a disease, but it is also the story of real people who made incredible sacrifices to stop it in its tracks.

Julie K. Silver, M.D.
Assistant Professor, Harvard Medical School
Department of Physical Medicine and Rehabilitation

Preface

Alcoholism, like all addictions, has long been considered a "social disease" caused by weakness of will, poor self-control, or lack of faith. Today, alcoholism is seen as a biological disease, one that has had great effects on mankind for centuries. From the Bible's frequent mention of alcohol abuse, to early medical recognition and the Temperance Movement, to the forming of Alcoholics Anonymous and Mothers Against Drunk Driving, to current advances in treatment and genetic research, alcoholism has existed and continues to cause significant problems for our health, our relationships, our jobs, our economy, and more. *Alcoholism* is designed to provide a balanced account of the disease in terms of its process and the impact it has had around the world, historically to present day. The text follows a timeline of alcoholism as first discussed in ancient times and traces the course of the disease as it has progressed, both socially and biologically. Written in a logical manner that allows the reader to follow the "life" of alcoholism, this text is to be used by students and others to learn about the disease in a different way and to gain understanding of the power that alcoholism can have on almost every aspect of life.

HOW TO USE THIS BOOK

Readers will receive information in a biographical timeline approach to alcoholism that can be read in a sequential manner that layers information onto the foundation of the previous chapter. The depth of knowledge and the span of information included make this book a perfect addition to an institution's library or to a personal collection. Students, along with others, will benefit from a thorough yet comprehensible analysis of the medical and social criteria of the disease. Each chapter covers its own independent subject matter and can be read separately with a sense of completeness, depending on the interests of the reader. Each chapter is divided into subchapters that contain relevant information on the topic at hand.

Chapter 1 begins with a historical look at alcoholism, from ancient myths surrounding the origin and meaning of alcohol to early medical pioneers who discovered and campaigned against alcohol abuse and its dire health effects. We follow the disease from its many mentions in The Bible through the first understandings of alcoholism as an actual disease. Chapter 2 looks at trends in alcohol use and defines alcoholism, providing distinctions between alcohol dependence and alcohol abuse. The signs and symptoms of alcoholism are explained, as well as common causes, risk factors, and health complications. Focus is given to the ongoing debate of whether alcoholism is moral or medical. Chapter 3 covers the complexities of diagnosing and treating alcoholism, from personal to professional screening tools and tactics to the significant impact of Alcoholics Anonymous. Treatment options and alternative therapies are discussed, as well as known barriers to treatment. Chapter 4 exposes the detrimental effects of alcoholism on our society. The reader will gain an understanding of how alcohol abuse touches our economy, our families, our laws, and our schools. Chapter 5 discusses problems linked to alcoholism, including violence and crime, sex-related troubles, multi-substance addiction, and nutritional deficiency. The text concludes with highlights of current research, genetic advances, new techniques, and political headway in the areas of alcoholism treatment and addiction therapy.

Acknowledgments

My sincere thanks to Dr. Julie Silver for this unique opportunity, Dr. Val Jones for her constant faith, Dr. Bruce Phariss for his exceptional advisement, and my team of editorial assistants—Stacy Friedman, Rich Majerus, Chris Gottschalk, and Sue Benedett—for making it all possible.

A special thanks to R.F.

Introduction

Throughout history, the moral condemnation of excessive alcohol use has run a parallel course to more acceptable forms of drinking. On one hand, religious leaders, temperance organizations, or recovery groups may devote considerable efforts to curbing alcohol use. On the other hand, others may see drinking as a normal or even healthy part of meals, celebrations, or religious ceremonies. In most people's minds, alcohol consumption itself is not disapproved of, but drinking to excess is usually seen as foolish, weak, or sinful.

Most characterizations of drunkenness have historically been unflattering, with all major world religions cautioning against the perils of heavy drinking to some degree. Many temperance movements viewed all forms of drinking as unacceptable, with even the most casual alcohol consumption leading inevitably to social ills like crime, poverty, and abandonment. Drinking was seen more as a moral weakness rather than a physical illness or physiological disorder. It wasn't until the mid-twentieth century that the theory of alcoholism as a disease became more accepted by the scientific community, with the World Health Organization defining alcoholism as one of a group of "dependence syndromes," in which the drinker has a relationship with alcohol by way of "impaired control over its use, persistent use despite harmful consequences, a higher priority given to drug use than to other activities and obligations, increased tolerance, and a physical withdrawal reaction when drug use is discontinued." Simply said, impaired control implies an involuntary state of addiction, not a moral weakness.

This reinforced the notion of alcoholics being helpless in their compulsion to drink.

The perception of alcoholism has evolved from sin to sickness, from a weakness of will to a legitimate public health issue. And although there isn't exact consensus about how to define alcoholism, most major providers of alcohol education and treatment, including Alcoholics Anonymous, the National Institute for Alcohol Abuse and Alcoholism, the American Medical Association, and the American Psychological Association, characterize alcoholism as a medical illness. Understandably, with drinking alcohol seeming like a voluntary activity, not everyone accepts the notion of alcoholism in this way, and the debate will likely continue for some time. For the purposes of this book, we look at alcohol dependence as a chronic disease, worthy of the same respect and support as any other disease.

1

Alcoholism, Historically

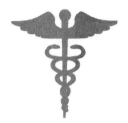

One that hath wine as a chain about his wits, such a one lives no life at all.
—Alcaeus 600 BCE

The history of alcoholism is in truth the history of alcohol itself, for people have been using and abusing alcohol since it was discovered thousands of years ago. Alcohol is presumably the first drug used by ancient man, and its effects, both enriching and damaging, have been well documented throughout the world for centuries. Alcohol transcended all boundaries in the ancient world—religiously, culturally, and geographically. In all parts of the world, alcohol was discovered and socially understood in similar ways.

AN ANCIENT MYTH

Alcaeus noted the detrimental side effects of alcohol dependence in Ancient Greece, as did Euripides in his ancient work *The Bacchae*. Euripides wrote that:

Dionysus came to Attica and was received as a guest by Icarius. Dionysus gave Icarius a branch of a grape vine and taught him wine-making. Icarius produced a batch of wine and, following the god's instructions, wished to share the gift with his fellow citizens. He offered the wine to some shepherds, and, once they tasted it, they found it delightful and began to drink copiously, without mixing it with water. But, as they began to feel its effects, they thought that Icarius had poisoned them, and they killed him. (Mikalson 2005, 60)

This ancient myth concludes with the establishing of festivals to worship Dionysus and Icarius. These festivals involve not only the drinking of wine, but also sacraments and libations of wine. Furthermore, the myth clearly shows the double-edged sword that Dionysus, the Greek god of wine, gave to mankind. On one hand, the use of wine brought joy and fellowship to Icarius' life as well as to the lives of the shepherds. On the other hand, the abuse of wine ultimately brought on the demise and death of Icarius in addition to casting a cloud of shame upon the shepherds. This myth shows that the Greeks understood that wine in moderation was socially beneficial and could help forge friendships, but at the same time they knew that wine in excess could quickly lead to the destruction of individuals and relationships. Thousands of years before the first medical professional spoke of alcoholism as a disease, ancient people believed that alcohol was a divine gift and understood that abusing wine was a human ailment.

ALCOHOL: A GIFT FROM THE GODS?

Most religions throughout the world took care to point out the differences between alcohol use and abuse, condoning the former and condemning the latter. The belief that wine was a gift from the gods and the reverence for its effects was in no way exclusive to Greece. In fact, it was almost universally accepted throughout ancient history. The Egyptian, Roman, and Mesopotamian cultures all held similar beliefs in their gods of wine, who were Osiris, Bacchus, and Siduri, respectively. Wine was one of two sources of necessary sustenance in the pagan times of the Roman Empire, with the other being bread. One of the earliest records of the use of alcohol, dating back to 3000 BCE in what was ancient Mesopotamian, comes from archeological findings that detail the use of beer in sacramental and religious rituals. The same clay tablets also provide ancient medicinal recipes using various combinations of wines and herbs.

The historic record of alcohol and alcohol abuse is bolstered by its frequent mention in the most popular book in the history of the world, the Bible. The Bible tells of how alcohol can make even the most pious person behave immorally or irrationally. This principle is illustrated when alcohol is abused by Noah, who becomes drunk and without reason curses his son Ham. Even Noah, who is seen by several religions as a rescuer, loses control and brings shame to his life by abusing alcohol.

Was alcohol truly a gift from the gods? This is an idea that was cited up until the early part of American history, and it is supported by the myth of Dionysus bringing wine-making to Thebes, as well as by the story of Jesus turning water

> **The Origins of Alcohol**
>
> While historians don't know exactly when alcohol was first created, they do know that it's been around throughout almost all of human history. Archaeologists have discovered beer jugs dating back to the Neolithic period, about 10,000 B.C., while Egyptian hieroglyphs as old as 3100 B.C. show that wine was enjoyed as far back as the first and second dynasties. According to the Old Testament, the earliest mentioned planter of vineyards was Noah, who was also the first person the Bible records as being drunk to the point of passing out.

into wine. If alcohol was not a magical gift from the gods, then how was it discovered? The answer may never be known, but it was indeed discovered, and discovered often. Almost every ancient civilization produced alcohol independently from one another.

EARLY "SPIRITS"

Ancient civilizations produced alcoholic beverages through a process called fermentation, a natural process that occurs when yeast interacts with sugars in fruits or grains, turning the sugar into alcohol. The fermentation of grapes produces wine, whereas the fermentation of grains, such as wheat and rice, produces beer. The ability for this process to occur naturally means that ancient people may have discovered fermentation by accident. With the right conditions, it would be possible for grapes out in the warm sun to ferment on their own without human intervention. Once the ancient people tasted what would have looked simply like rotten grapes, they would have discovered the unique and mystical effects of fermented fruits. It is logical to assume that they then went on to purposefully produce similar substances in large quantities.

In this way, ancient people began to understand the production of alcohol in addition to what its mystical effects were, but they did not completely comprehend the science behind its production or its interaction with the body. Since the creation of wine and beer could not be scientifically explained at that time, ancient people used myth to justify its existence.

It wasn't until the 10th century that alcohol was understood more completely. At that time, the process of distillation was documented at a medical school in Salerno, Italy. Distillation is an unnatural process that is performed by humans on a liquid that has already been fermented. The alcohol in the fermented mixture is brought to a boil and turned into steam, which travels through piping to a colder container, where the steam is condensed back into a liquid. Since alcohol boils at a low temperature, most of what is transferred into the colder container is pure alcohol, making distilled liquor up to 15 times more potent than beer. Fermented alcohol, which has been consumed for the better part of history, has an alcohol content of less than 14 percent, whereas distilled liquor can contain as much as 90 percent alcohol.

These extremely potent alcoholic beverages were termed "spirits" because they contained the spirit of the wine. The spirit of wine, which is the alcohol created through fermentation, is greatly condensed in the production of hard liquor, such as brandy or whiskey, so the liquor does contain the essence of the original wine. Early Middle Eastern cultures discovered how to distill what they called "al kohl," from which the modern term "alcohol" is derived. *Al kohl* originally meant a finely ground powder, which was often used in makeup, but eventually came to mean any substance that was extracted from another, especially alcohol. This new form of distilled alcohol was much more intoxicating and deadening to the body's senses than wine and beer, and as a result was widely used as a pain medication.

ALCOHOL AS MEDICINE

Give strong drink unto him who is ready to perish, and wine unto those that be of heavy heart. Let him drink, and forget his poverty, and remember his misery no more.

—Book of Proverbs

Early Americans were God-fearing people for the most part, especially since many of them came to the colonies in order to escape religious persecution. Therefore, many Americans followed the Bible almost word for word. When the Bible said "drink," they drank—and probably more than was intended by the Book of Proverbs. There is evidence of medical practitioners giving alcohol as a primitive painkiller to those who were extremely ill. Many men and women drank to drown their sorrows, a common practice still seen today. In early American history, people drank for all reasons. Any social event was a just cause for indulgence, such as weddings, funerals, elections, or the construction of a new building.

Alcohol use was so prevalent and accepted that the substance was termed aqua vitae, or "water of life." It was thought to increase one's health and vitality. During westward expansion in America, for example, it was believed that alcoholic beverages gave working men the extra strength they needed to perform hard labor, and supervisors often paid laborers with alcohol. At that time, alcohol was viewed with great esteem and even thought to be a medical cure-all.

The view of alcohol as an element of health was held long before the early settlers landed on the eastern shore of America. One of the earliest references to alcohol being used as medicine is present on a cuneiform tablet—one of the earliest forms of written expression—dating from 2200 BCE, on which beer is recommended as a tonic for lactating women. This is an interesting prescription for alcohol, considering what the medical community today knows about the effects of alcohol on fetal and infant brain development. However, even modern medicine, with all of its advances in research and technology, was unaware of and did not acknowledge fetal alcohol syndrome (FAS) until the 1970s.

The connection between mothers, children, and alcohol has fascinated medical professionals throughout history. In the 1700s, Thomas Trotter, a Scottish physician, hypothesized that a mother who stops breastfeeding her child too early will raise the child's chance of becoming an alcoholic later in life. Trotter's hypothesis was confirmed in the 1960s by scientists at the Institute of Preventive Medicine in Copenhagen, Denmark. At that time, babies were often given small amounts of alcohol in their bottles to soothe them, while young children were given alcohol to become accustomed to its effects. From birth, people were acquiring a taste for alcohol.

This practice has greatly changed in America, but it may have changed more recently than many people think. Young Americans regularly consumed alcohol at home well into the 20th century. Many other practices and beliefs surrounding alcohol have changed in recent history as the medical and scientific knowledge of alcohol has evolved. For instance, in early America women would drink much less in public than they do today. This is because women were expected to be especially conscious of their social behavior in order to remain "lady-like." However, this social persona often led women to drink alcohol-based medicines for their health. Many who regarded spirits as "vulgar" happily downed a highly alcoholic cordial or stomach elixir (Rorabaugh 1979). It was harder for women to drink enough to become drunk because of these social stipulations. As a result, they drank behind closed doors and used the supposed medical benefits of alcohol to justify using and abusing it. Women were not the only ones to use medicine as an excuse to drink. This was common practice for both sexes throughout history. Women were simply socially compelled to claim medicinal reasons more often.

In fact, the medicinal cover-up of alcohol consumption is a problem that has persisted throughout American history. Prohibition triggered a significant increase in the number of doctors and drugstores applying for licenses to sell medicinal liquor. The supposed medicinal qualities of alcohol were a mask for alcohol use that Americans called on whenever they saw necessary.

THE CHURCH AND ALCOHOL ABUSE

Even more connected to alcohol in early America was another unsuspected culprit for alcohol abuse: the church. Alcohol was not just considered the "water of life," but the "the good creature of God" as well. The Puritans were the only early American religious group that outlawed drunkenness, but even this religion, which is still notorious for its strictness with alcohol, allowed drinking.

The clergy were among the biggest alcohol indulgers in America from the late 1700s until the mid-1800s. In those days, clergymen made house calls to various parishioners. A clergyman would make many of these house calls in a day and would have at least one drink at each home as part of the meeting ritual. According to an advocate of temperance in 1857, 50 percent of the clergy died drunkards (Rorabaugh 1979). Drinking was so prominent among the clergy that taverns often were constructed next to churches to accommodate clergymen between services. Any religious ceremony turned into an opportunity to indulge in alcohol at the local tavern, so it was simply good business to build a tavern next to a church.

In the middle of the 19th century, the religious voice in early America slowly began to shift from that of hardy drinkers to staunch advocates of temperance because of the social ills that they began to attribute to alcohol abuse. Temperance advocates began to use religion to combat excessive drinking as the medical approach to the ills of alcohol consumption promoted by Trotter proved to be ineffective at that time in history. Religious leaders started to attack the idea that alcohol was "the good creature of God," saying that alcohol is different than what God put here and that man created alcohol. They claimed that alcohol was an evil creation of man prompted by the Devil, not a divine gift from God. As a result, liquor was blamed for all social ills, and church leaders began to make moral appeals to their followers in order to curb the social problems that they saw stemming from alcohol abuse. Mark Matthews, a reverend in Seattle, went as far as to say that:

> The saloon is the most fiendish, corrupt, hell-soaked institution that ever crawled out of the slime of the eternal pit. It takes your sweet innocent daughter, robs her of her virtue, and transforms her into a brazen, wanton harlot. It is the open sore of this land. (Behr 1996)

Reverend Justin Edwards was one of several clergymen who took a different approach to combating intemperance by creating a physical fear in his followers who abused alcohol. He propagated the idea that alcohol abuse could cause people to spontaneously combust, telling his followers to "take the blood of a drunkard, from his head, or his liver, and distill it. It has actually been taken from the brain, strong enough, on application of fire, to burn" (Behr 1996). As religious fervor replaced the medical and scientific appeals for temperance, which were ineffective at the time, abstinence from alcohol use became associated with salvation and drunkenness with damnation. Even Benjamin Franklin said that drinking had caused an increase in "swearing, poverty, and the distaste for religion" (Behr 1996).

ALCOHOL IN COLONIAL TIMES AND EARLY AMERICA

Is it not mortifying . . . that we, Americans, should exceed all other . . . people in the world in this degrading, beastly vice of intemperance?

—John Adams

On the surface there appears to be a consensus among the Founding Fathers of our country that excessive drinking was damaging the fabric of the nation. However, many were heavy drinkers themselves. For example, George Washington spent one-fourth of his personal expenses on booze during his first months in the presidency, and James Madison reportedly drank a pint of whiskey before breakfast. Even John Adams began his days with a draft of hard cider, though he said this in his campaign against alcohol:

> I am fired with a zeal amounting to enthusiasm against ardent spirits, the multiplication of taverns, retailer, dram-shops and tippling houses, grieved to the heart to see the number of idlers, thieves, Sots and consumptive patients made for the physician in these infamous seminaries. (Behr 1996)

The problem of alcohol abuse in America goes back before the Founding Fathers even set foot on American soil. The majority of early settlers were heavy drinkers. The pilgrims aboard the Mayflower chose to land at Plymouth Rock in part because they were running out of beer. They were actually headed for Virginia, but changed course because of storms. Justifying their choice to settle at Plymouth Rock, one pilgrim said: "We could not take time for further search or consideration, our victuals [supplies] being much spent, especially our beer" (Beyer 2003). Many things were brought to America by the pilgrims, a passion for alcohol included.

About 100 years after the pilgrims arrived in America, the gin epidemic struck England in the 1720s. England had accumulated a negative trade balance that compelled it to turn inward for more industrial production. This fact, combined with a significant drop in grain prices, led to mass production of gin, which burst on the scene in large quantities and was often abused by the lower and working classes. British soldiers, for example, were given two pounds of bread, one pound of meat, and four pints of beer daily. Beer was clearly the drink of choice as well as the daily drink of the British army, whereas the Colonial army provided its soldiers with a daily ration of four ounces of whiskey or rum.

Colonial Americans were aligned with their British counterparts when it came to drinking. Alcohol became so commonplace in Colonial American that it infiltrated courtroom trials, what were supposed to be the most just of meetings. In pre-independence times, the colonies' judges were so frequently drunk at the bench that heavy fines were instituted for those proved incapable during court proceedings (Behr 1996). These are the very same judges that were in charge of imposing penalties on excessive drinkers. The judges were supposed to help enforce laws concerning the amount of alcohol that could be served to each patron at a tavern and how long these patrons could remain at a tavern. However, the rules were rarely enforced (Behr 1996). The laws may have been ignored or difficult to enforce because the judges were as intoxicated as the defendants.

Drinking was so prominent in the judicial system that in Virginia, where the law allowed only one tavern per county, a drinking place was most often adjoined to the courthouse. Before trials, it was common for defendants, attorneys, judges, and jurymen to gather there to drink, and sometimes matters were settled "out-of-court" (Rorabaugh 1979). When the penalties for excessive public drunkenness were enforced, they were often more of a social penalty opposed to a stay in jail or a fine. For instance, in Massachusetts, habitual offenders were exposed to public ridicule and made to wear shirts inscribed with a large "D" or the word "Drunkard" (Behr 1996). Considering how accepted drinking was at this time in American history, this was likely viewed as a minimal penalty.

After all, drinking alcohol in the 18th century was safer than drinking water. The quality of water was erratic and ranged from drinkable to horribly contaminated. Many bouts of illness were traced to water consumption. On the other hand, since the water used to distill spirits was boiled, it was essentially purified. Alcohol in the spirits killed the vast majority of remaining bacteria, making alcohol significantly more consistent in quality than water. In 1760, the average American consumed 3.7 gallons of alcoholic spirits. This is not to say that every American was a drunkard. Statistics show that one-eighth of the population drank two-thirds of the hard liquor consumed in the United States, which means that a small group of Americans drank most of the liquor (Rorabaugh 1979).

Most of this alcohol was drunk at home, and drinking at the tavern became a certain right of passage for young American men. Young adolescent teens would stake their claim on manhood by going out to the local tavern with their fathers. There was no official drinking age, so the age at which a young man began going to the tavern was a matter of debate between him and his father. It seems to have happened sooner rather than later, as there are accounts of boys as young as 12 years of age being present at taverns with their fathers. Parents justified drinking at this age with the belief that allowing young people to consume alcohol in a supervised environment would reduce excessive consumption later in life. Apparently, this approach did not work because Americans would drink at any time, at any place, and on any occasion.

The natural tendency of Americans to consume alcohol excessively became so evident that visitors to the United States began to take notice. For example, the Scotsman Peter Neilson commented that the Americans were "in a certain degree seasoned" when it came to drinking (Rorabaugh 1979). Neilson's observation was backed by statistics showing that during the early nineteenth century Americans drank more than the English, Irish, or Prussians, and about the same as the Scots and French, but less than the Swedes (Rorabaugh 1979). The drinking prowess of Americans was so evident that it was clearly recognized by both international visitors and even those who had never set foot on American soil.

This is not to say that the excessive drinking of Americans was not recognized internally by American citizens themselves. At the time when those young teens who went to the taverns with their fathers in the early days of American Independence would have been older adults, the *Old American Encyclopedia* published the following excerpt about pre-independence drinking:

> A fashion at the South was to take a glass of whiskey, flavoured with mint, soon after waking. . . . At eleven o'clock, while mixtures, under various peculiar names—sling, toddy, flip—solicited the appetite . . . the offices of professional men and wonting rooms dismissed their occupants for a half hour to regale themselves at a neighbor's or a coffee-house with punch. . . . At the dinner hour . . . whiskey and water . . . introduced the feast; whiskey or brandy and water helped it thought and whiskey or brandy without water secured its safe digestion. . . . Rum, seasoned with cherries, protected against the cold; rum, made astringent with peach-nuts, concluded the repast at the confectioner's; rum, made nutritious with milk, prepared for the maternal office. (Behr 1996)

According to this passage, it appears that the standard was at least seven drinks a day: one before breakfast, a couple in the afternoon, and a few more with dinner. Americans knew they drank at lot. However, what would now be considered excessive consumption was not seen as a problem at that point in American history. The first American to take a scientific approach to the eradication of excessive consumption was the Surgeon General of the Colonial Army, Dr. Benjamin Rush. Unfortunately, Rush's efforts were largely unsuccessful, and his thoughts were often dismissed because of the prevalence of alcohol in American culture.

FROM SIN TO SICKNESS: MEDICAL PIONEERS

> *In folly, [alcohol] causes him to resemble a calf; in stupidity, an ass; in roaring, a mad bull; in quarreling and fighting, a dog; in cruelty, a tiger; in fetor, a skunk; in filthiness, a hog; and in obscenity, a he-goat.*
>
> —Dr. Benjamin Rush

Dr. Benjamin Rush's commentary on alcohol may sound absurd if it were to be heard from a practitioner of modern medicine. One must remember, however, that Rush was not fighting against scientifically proven benefits of alcohol, but rather against the psychological and moral beliefs in the power of a drug. Accordingly, Dr. Rush took an extreme approach to his writings about the detrimental effects of alcohol, and often strayed from scientific arguments to moral ones in order to reach the consciousness of the American people.

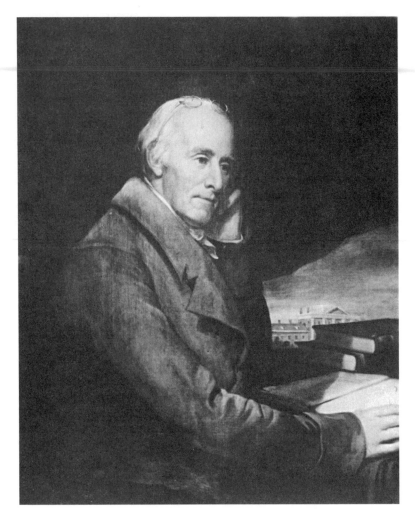

Figure 1.1 Dr. Benjamin Rush, the Surgeon General of the Colonial Army, was a leader in the early campaign against alcoholism and the first American to scientifically declare excessive alcohol use as unhealthy. [Courtesy of National Archives, photo no. NWDNS-148-CP-0200]

Dr. Rush was not alone in his fight against the idea that alcohol "could cure cold, fevers, snakebites, frosted toes, and broken legs, and as relaxants that would relieve depression, reduce tension, and enable hardworking laborers to enjoy a moment of happy, frivolous camaraderie" (Rorabaugh 1979). He and his colleagues Nathaniel Ames, Dr. Ann Preston, and Dr. Thomas Trotter may have jump-started the temperance movement, but it took more than 100 more years for the idea that alcohol was harmful to the human body to be accepted.

Nathaniel Ames was the first American to associate alcohol with side effects that were harmful to the human body. In the 1750s, he said that "Strong Waters were formerly used only by the Direction of Physicians; but now Mechanicks drink Rum like Fountain-Water, and they can infinitely better endure it than the idle . . . DEATH is in the bottom of the cup of every one" (Lee 1963). Like Dr. Rush, Ames took an extreme approach to combating intemperance in America. He also made a key observation that hard liquor was first used for medicinal purposes and from that point it spiraled out of control. This would prove to be an issue that the United States would revisit over 170 years later when Congress held debates on the acceptability of "medicinal beer" during Prohibition.

Dr. Ann Preston was born to a Quaker minister in 1813, the year Dr. Rush died. She was a prominent member of the Clarkson Anti-Slavery Society and the temperance movement. Her struggle as a woman to become a doctor in the 19th century created a desire in her to help others fight for equal rights, and she was one of the pioneers who meshed the temperance movement with the movement for women's rights.

Dr. Thomas Trotter, a prestigious physician to the Channel fleet and a surgeon in the Royal Navy, fought the same fight in Scotland as Dr. Rush did in America. Dr. Trotter and Dr. Rush were contemporaries writing in the same period for the same cause. Dr. Trotter published his first work against excessive alcohol consumption titled "Thesis De Ebrietate" in 1788, and an updated version titled "An Essay on Drunkenness" followed in 1804. In his writing, Dr. Trotter presented alcohol abuse as a disease for the first time in medical history.

Dr. Rush, who graduated from Princeton University at 15 years of age, is one of the lesser-known Founding Fathers of America. He was, however, the most prestigious of the doctors in the early campaign against alcoholism, largely because of his political prowess and connections. Shortly after he signed the Declaration of Independence, Dr. Rush published *An Inquiry into the Effects of Spirituous Liquors on the Human Body and Mind,* which sold 170,000 copies. In this work, which has been cited throughout American history, Dr. Rush catalogued liquor's defects, saying that it protected against neither hot nor cold weather and caused numerous illnesses, including stomach sickness, vomiting, hand tremors, dropsy, liver disorders, madness, palsy, apoplexy, and epilepsy (Rorabaugh 1979). Dr. Rush went against the popular trend in America by saying that alcohol was not a healthy stimulant and that it had no health benefit. In order to illustrate his point more clearly, Dr. Rush included the "Moral and Physical Thermometer of Intemperance" along with his essay. The "Thermometer" lists beverages in order from the most temperate to the most intemperate, and indicates the effects that correspond with the consumption of each beverage. Dr. Rush lists the most temperate beverages as water, milk, and small amounts of beer, and says that they lead to health, wealth, serenity of the mind, reputation, long life, and happiness. Conversely, Dr. Rush lists the most intemperate beverages as gin, brandy, and rum, and says that they lead to burglary, murder, madness, and apoplexy. The title of Dr. Rush's "Thermometer,", not to mention the effects and consequences he lists, clearly show how he chose to cross back and forth between science and moral arguments concerning intemperance.

This being said, Dr. Rush did not want to ban alcohol. He only saw hard liquor as the problem, not wine and beer. As a cure for liquor abuse, Dr. Rush proposed mixing wine with opium to calm down the alcoholic until he or she was free from the effects of hard alcohol. As was common for advocates in Dr. Rush's time, he took on many causes, not just hard liquor. Dr. Rush attacked the use of tobacco, was an active antislavery advocate, and campaigned for the better treatment of people with mental illness (Rorabaugh 1979). Dr. Rush's passions for temperance and freedom closely parallel those of Frederick Douglass, one of the most famous advocates in American history. In a speech in Ireland, Douglass said, "I believe, Mr. President, that if we could but make the world sober, we would have no slavery. I believe that if the slaveholder would be sober for a moment, he would consider the sinfulness of his position" (Douglass 1845). Dr. Rush provided the foundation for such statements with his "Thermometer," which was considered factual and demonstrated that liquor not only clouds the mind but leads to worse vices.

The most prominent of Dr. Rush's causes was his campaign for those suffering from mental illness. Dr. Rush proposed several innovations for both the understanding of mental illnesses and the treatment of people suffering from such illnesses. Dr. Rush's convictions led him to be one of the few to recognize that mental illness could be diagnosed, classified, and treated (Pennsylvania Health System). His understanding of the mind and mental illness is likely why Dr. Rush was the first American to view alcoholism as a disease rather than a choice.

2

Alcohol Use and Abuse

With all of the serious risks linked to alcohol, why do people drink at all? Some reasons are obvious: Drinking makes many people feel good. Alcohol consumption affects the mechanism of certain brain chemicals called neurotransmitters, including:

- **Gamma-amino butyric acid (GABA).** This neurotransmitter is responsible for inhibiting brain activity. Alcohol stimulates the brain's GABA receptors, which is why many people find it relaxing to drink.
- **Dopamine.** Alcohol and many other addictive substances increase the levels of this chemical in the brain, which is associated with pleasurable sensations that follow experiences like eating and sex. When someone drinks, the resulting surplus of dopamine is what provides the euphoric feeling associated with being intoxicated, and it plays an important role in the emergence of alcohol addiction.
- **Serotonin.** An imbalance of this neurotransmitter is involved in mood disorders like depression and anxiety. Some research suggests that alcohol may increase the brain's serotonin activity, which can either elevate or depress mood, depending on the person drinking. This alteration of serotonin activity may also contribute to withdrawal symptoms of sleeplessness and anxiety. Serotonin also increases the activity of GABA and

dopamine, triggering other effects, such as memory problems, confusion, and problems concentrating.

The immediate effects of altering these neurotransmitters leads to the pleasant aspects of drinking, such as feeling happy, relaxed, aroused, or intoxicated. It can also cause people to lose their inhibitions, experience exaggerated emotions, or become hostile and uptight. It depends on each individual's neurological response to alcohol. Pleasant effects aside, drinking may have more complicated and sometimes hidden consequences, including:

- **Loneliness or grief.** Some people use alcohol as a way to cope with a death, divorce, or other life event. Others want to escape feelings of being lonely or sad, and find solace by drinking rather than getting to the root of their troubling emotions.
- **Stress.** Everyday pressures can for example, cause some people to turn to alcohol to relieve stress. Military veterans, or other people who suffer from post-traumatic stress disorder sometimes find drinking to be a temporary shortcut to feeling calm.
- **Psychological issues.** For people who struggle with depression, anxiety, or problems with self-esteem, drinking may be a way to steady their nerves or stave off the effects of certain psychological imbalances.
- **Peer behavior.** This common reason for drinking is a compelling one for young people, who may be tempted or even pressured by their peers' behavior around alcohol. Teenagers who are curious about drinking may find it easier to pick up that first beer if their friends are encouraging them to do so.
- **Home life.** Kids in troubled homes or an environment of heavy alcohol use are more likely to develop drinking problems. Other difficulties, such as depression or violence in the home, also increase a child's risk of alcohol abuse in the long term. However, not every young person in such a situation is destined to become a problem drinker.

HOW MUCH IS TOO MUCH? A LOOK AT BLOOD ALCOHOL

In determining how much someone has to drink in order to feel alcohol's intoxicating effects, no discussion would be complete without exploring the idea of blood alcohol levels. Most people have heard the phrase blood alcohol levels (BAL), or blood alcohol content (BAC)—one of the few tangible ways to measure how much alcohol is in someone's system. Police officers and other law enforcement officials use blood alcohol levels to determine how much a driver has had to drink. In hospitals, emergency-room physicians may measure a person's blood alcohol levels to get a sense for how much he or she has had to drink.

> **How Addictive Is Alcohol?**
>
> According to a study commissioned by the National Institute on Drug Abuse, alcohol is one of the more addictive drugs. While it creates less dependence in the user than nicotine, heroin, or cocaine, alcohol's withdrawal symptoms are worse. Alcohol is more addictive than marijuana.

But what is blood alcohol level a measure of exactly? Simply put, it is the amount of alcohol concentration in the blood, which is determined by the weight of alcohol (in grams) per 100 milliliters (mL), or deciliter, in the blood. For example, a blood alcohol level of 0.07 percent means that the person has 70 milligrams (or 4/1000th of a gram) of alcohol in their system per deciliter of blood. Something measured in milligrams may not seem like a large amount, but it doesn't take many milligrams of alcohol for disastrous effects to occur. A blood alcohol level of 0.30 percent, for example, can cause coma or death. Since alcohol is absorbed into the blood very quickly after being consumed, it doesn't take long for a person's blood alcohol levels to be affected by drinking.

Factors Affecting Blood Alcohol Levels

Blood alcohol levels are influenced by many factors, which is why drinking affects different people in different ways. As one might guess, a big person who has eaten a meal before drinking will not absorb alcohol in the same way as a small person drinking on an empty stomach.

Weight

In most cases, weight is the primary factor affecting blood alcohol levels. To most people this is obvious: The more a person weighs, the more body mass he or she has to absorb the alcohol and become affected by drinking.

Sex

A person's sex can determine how their blood alcohol levels will be affected by drinking. Men and women metabolize alcohol differently, even if they are the same size, and this plays a role in how each experiences alcohol's effects. The main reason is that men's bodies generally contain a higher percentage of water than women's bodies do—61 percent for the average man versus 52 percent for the average woman—and this helps dilute the absorption of alcohol. Women also have lower amounts of the enzyme alcohol dehydrogenase, a substance used by the liver to metabolize alcohol, so females break down alcohol more slowly.

Hormonal factors can also influence the effects of drinking for women, particularly premenstrual hormones, which can increase the likelihood of a woman becoming intoxicated. The hormonal ingredients in birth control pills or estrogen supplements may decrease the rate that a woman eliminates alcohol from her body.

Additionally, women experience different, and sometimes more severe, long-term health effects from drinking than men do, including brain and liver damage, high blood pressure, cirrhosis, heart disease, and social effects, such as victimization and car accidents.

Number of Drinks and Rate of Drinking

Blood alcohol levels aren't just affected by how many drinks a person consumes, but how many he or she has per hour. The National Highway Traffic Safety Administration (NHTSA) estimates that, in most people, the liver can safely metabolize one drink per hour, although this may not be true for everyone. Someone who has never had alcohol may become tipsy after just one drink. Conversely, a person who has developed a high tolerance for alcohol may not feel the effects of more than one drink per hour.

In this one-drink-per-hour calculation, the NHTSA counts one drink as a 12-ounce can of beer, a 5-ounce glass of wine, or a 1.5-ounce serving of liquor (such as vodka or gin). People who play drinking games that involve chugging alcohol or doing shots, for example, will feel alcohol's effects more quickly and put themselves at higher risk for problems related to binge drinking (more on that later).

Other Factors

Weight, sex, and rate of drinking are the most common factors affecting blood alcohol levels, but it can also be affected by other circumstances as well, such as:

- How much the drinker has had to eat—having food in the stomach slows down alcohol absorption and, therefore, lowers the rate of blood alcohol increase. The food doesn't actually "soak up" the alcohol—it merely delays its effects.
- Whether the drink was carbonated or not—bubbly beverages contain carbon dioxide (CO_2), which causes the alcohol to be absorbed more quickly, creating a more rapid rise in blood alcohol levels. This explains why drinks such as champagne seem to go to a person's head more readily than their noncarbonated counterparts, such as wine or fruity cocktails.

- Temperature—warm alcoholic drinks (such as Irish coffee) are absorbed more rapidly than cooler beverages.
- Age—for various reasons, adolescents and senior citizens may absorb alcohol differently than the rest of the population, experiencing higher BALs and, therefore, being more vulnerable to alcohol's effects.
- Medications—certain medications, such as antianxiety drugs, can interact with alcohol and increase its effects.

Estimating Blood Alcohol Levels

Anyone who wants to estimate how drinking will affect his or her own blood alcohol levels can find this information on the Internet, which features dozens of free BAL calculation tools. These tools generally use a person's weight, sex, and number of drinks per hour to calculate BAL. Typing "BAL calculator" into an Internet search engine will provide a list of such calculators.

However, it's important to remember that BAL calculators are just tools for estimating blood alcohol levels and shouldn't be used to determine how much alcohol is "safe" to drink. For some people, even small amounts of alcohol can cause problems with judgment that make it unsafe to drive or make good decisions.

Blood Alcohol Levels, Drunk Driving, and Unsafe Behavior

What does it mean to know the percentage of alcohol in a person's blood, whether it's 0.03 percent or 0.15 percent? How can such a small amount of alcohol affect someone? To put such percentages into a more meaningful light, it may be helpful to consider the blood alcohol measurement that all 50 U.S. states have deemed criminally unsafe for driving: 0.08 percent. Anyone at this percentage or higher is considered to be too dangerously affected by drinking to operate a car safely and will be charged with driving under the influence of alcohol (DUI) or driving while intoxicated (DWI). Depending on the state, the consequences of a DUI or DWI can include a revoked license, community service, special alcohol-awareness classes, aversion therapy, or an impounded vehicle. But the consequences of driving under the influence—car crashes, injury, death—can be much more serious than those punishments.

Furthermore, even moderate drinking can cause problems for people behind the wheel, especially younger and newer drivers, who are still getting used to the rules of the road and the feel of the car, and who may feel more social pressure to drink and drive or ride in a car with someone who has been drinking. Young people may also be more strongly affected by alcohol, in which case even a 0.02 percent BAL could trigger dangerous lapses in judgment. In 2006, the Centers for Disease Control and Prevention reported that 19 percent of all fatally injured 16-to-20-year-old drivers had been drinking, with blood alcohol at a variety of levels.

Many people associate drunk drivers with an image of someone who is slurring their words, stumbling, and unable to stand up. While this image is accurate for many dangerously inebriated motorists, a person doesn't need to feel or appear drunk to be impaired by moderate drinking. He or she can easily be affected even when driving well within the legal blood alcohol limit. The National Highway Transportation Safety Administration reported in 1997 that 18 percent of fatally injured drivers had blood alcohol levels below the legal limit. Low BALs can cause attention difficulties, slowed reaction times, and impaired decision-making abilities, all of which increase the chances of a crash. For this reason, it might be more accurate to refer to the crime of drunk driving as alcohol-impaired driving.

Dangers of high blood alcohol levels are certainly not limited to driving. The Johns Hopkins School of Public Health published a study that identified alcohol as a leading cause of many types of fatal injuries, including fires and burns, frostbite and hypothermia, suicide, drowning, alcohol poisoning caused by binge drinking, and interactions with standard medications such as over-the-counter painkillers.

Pleasurable Effects of Alcohol: Moderation Is Key

In a safe, adult social setting, with designated drivers and other sensible measures in place, moderate drinking can be a pleasurable activity with many relaxing effects. The U.S. Department of Health and Human Services defines moderate drinking as a maximum of one drink per day for women and two per day for men. In the right amounts, alcohol can help a person relax and engage more easily in social situations, decrease stress, and promote carefree feelings. Moderate drinking has even been associated with certain health benefits such as lowered risk of heart attack and stroke. The National Institute on Alcohol Abuse and Alcoholism reported that among the elderly, moderate drinking was associated with increased appetite, improved bowel function, and elevated mood (although guidelines for maximum alcohol consumption for the elderly are lower than those for the general population).

The key idea among these benefits is moderation. Once a person passes the threshold from light drinking to heavy consumption, the effects of alcohol change from euphoric to unpleasant or dangerous. Research shows that the desired effects of alcohol usually occur with blood alcohol levels between 0.04 and 0.05. A 2009 study published in the journal *Alcoholism: Clinical & Experimental Research* found that the beta-endorphins ("feel-good" brain chemicals) associated with light or moderate drinking tapered off after a couple drinks, and anything beyond this level of alcohol consumption led to the more familiar outcomes of drinking: anxiety, stupor, amnesia, and increased aggression, among other effects. In fact, the study's authors advised that anyone who doesn't feel the pleasurable effects of alcohol after two drinks (or one drink for women) should stop drinking.

In addition, drinking beyond the moderate level increases the risk of alcohol-related problems, such as the impaired judgment that leads to drunk driving, violence, and unintended sexual encounters. Many college students who engage in binge drinking unfortunately become aware of the consequences of these acts.

Excessive Alcohol and Younger Drinkers

Why is it that some people are able to drink at a slower pace to experience alcohol's pleasant effects without getting drunk, while others plunge headfirst into the sloppier habits of heavy drinking? For one thing, some drinkers are more genetically, biologically, or socially predisposed to become addicted to alcohol. This is why two people may engage in the same drinking habits, but only one may emerge with a problem. But while that may explain the behavior of an alcoholic, it doesn't explain the behavior of younger drinkers, such as those in college, who may be abusing alcohol but aren't full-blown addicts yet.

Binge drinking among adolescents and college students remains an alarmingly common occurrence. The 2005 National Survey on Drug Use and Health estimated that almost 7.2 million underage drinkers drank enough to be considered binge drinkers—consuming more than four drinks on one occasion for females, and more than five drinks on one occasion for males. The reasons for excessive drinking are numerous among young people:

- **Relieving social awkwardness**—drinking can help shy people open up and feel more comfortable in social settings.
- **Brain not fully mature yet**—because the human brain is not fully developed until the age of 25, the area of the brain responsible for moderation isn't mature in most young drinkers.
- **Peer pressure**—this age-old social dynamic is a common culprit for many teen behaviors, and drinking is among the most common ways many young people believe they must fit in, feeling like they have to go along with others.
- **Lack of experience and judgment around alcohol**—without knowing the effects of alcohol, many young people overindulge, thinking that if one drink produces a light buzz, then two or three more will certainly be a harmless way to keep that happy feeling going.
- **Feeling immortal**—many adolescents have a hard time imagining anything unfortunate happening to them and may not be able to envision the dangerous effects of alcohol. And since many young people rebound easily from alcohol's effects (sleep deprivation, hangovers, and other ills), their feelings of immortality may be even stronger.
- **Impressing others**—a common show of teen bravado is to "drink someone under the table."

When Blood Alcohol Is Too High

The faster and more excessively a person drinks, the greater the chance of dangerous consequences. Although the effects of different blood alcohol levels vary and are hard to predict for each individual, guidelines show how the body is affected at each level.

When Blood Alcohol Is Too High

0.02 to 0.03
    Mild euphoria
    Coordination usually intact
    Effects of alcohol hard to detect
    May impair ability to drive
    Legally intoxicated for underage drinkers in some U.S. states
0.04 to 0.07
    Relaxation
    Lowered inhibitions
    Feeling of warmth
    Euphoria
    Problems with memory
    Slower reaction times
    Exaggerated emotion and behavior
    Tendency to keep drinking
    Decreased caution
0.08 to 0.09
    Slurred speech
    Problems with balance
    Reaction times and motor skills noticeably affected
    Mood swings
    Unable to recognize drunkenness
    False sense of confidence
    Unreliable judgment and self-control
    Legally drunk in all U.S. states   *(continued)*

- **Drinking games**—many high school and college students break the ice at social gatherings by engaging in this common pastime.
- **Alleviate pressure**—overscheduled adolescents may turn to excessive drinking to unwind from the demands of school, work, or social pressures.
- **Limited access to alcohol**—since they can't buy it themselves, underage drinkers may chug alcohol whenever they can get it.
- **Experimenting**—teens and adolescents are naturally curious about alcohol and other mood-altering substances, and they may drink excessively just to know what it feels like.

When Blood Alcohol Is Too High (*continued*)

0.10 to 0.12
  Obvious impairment of balance and coordination
  Loss of judgment and mental abilities
  Severely slurred speech
0.13 to 0.16
  Blurred vision
  Possible need for medical help
  Major problems with speech, balance, mental ability,
0.17 to 0.30
  Passing out
  Barely conscious
  Probably in need of medical attention
  Possibly comatose
  Complete loss of motor control
0.31 to 0.60
  Unconsciousness
  Coma
  Severe danger of death by alcohol poisoning

Binge Drinking and Alcohol Poisoning

Among the many problems arising from binge drinking, which include compromised judgment, risk of violence, high blood pressure, and accidents, none is more serious than alcohol poisoning. This is a dangerous condition that can be thought of as an alcohol overdose—too much drinking at once. When this happens, the overabundance of alcohol in the drinker's system dampens the nerves in the body that control breathing, which can lead to dangerously slow heart rhythms and death. Or it may inhibit the gag reflex, in which case the person could choke to death if he or she happened to vomit from too much drinking.

Alcohol poisoning is a particularly common problem on college campuses, where binge-drinking is part of many social events. There is no standard amount of alcohol that causes this potentially fatal condition, so each person's threshold is different. Since excessive drinking often causes a person to lose consciousness or "pass out," the symptoms of alcohol poisoning can go unnoticed if a drunk person's friends decide to let him or her "sleep it off." Most of the time, letting the person sleep until the alcohol's effects wear off is a safe decision, but if the person has alcohol poisoning, this decision can be fatal. Blood alcohol levels can continue to rise in a person who has lost consciousness, even after he or she stops drinking, possibly reaching lethal levels. Therefore, it's important to know the signs of alcohol poisoning. A person could be in danger if he or she:

out and cannot be awakened.
...its while unconscious and is not awakened by it.
...las cold, clammy, and pale or bluish skin.
• Is breathing very slowly—fewer than nine times per minute or with 10 seconds between breaths.

If you notice any of these signs, call 9-1-1 immediately, and don't worry about embarrassment, legal issues, or the person getting mad at you—this is a potentially life-threatening situation that always calls for emergency measures. While waiting for help to arrive, do not leave the person alone. Turn the person on their side to prevent choking, and try to wake them up periodically.

Myths About "Sobering Up"

There are a lot of misconceptions on the subject of what to do when someone is dangerously drunk. Common myths include:

- **Coffee**. Having caffeine may wake up a drunk person a little bit, but it won't lower blood alcohol levels or improve that person's ability to function or drive.
- **Cold shower**. Again, this may make the person more alert temporarily, but it won't affect blood alcohol levels.
- **Eating**. Having food before drinking will slow down the rate at which the body absorbs alcohol and how quickly the person feels alcohol's effects but once someone is intoxicated, the body has already absorbed the alcohol. Eating will have no effect at that point.
- **Walking or exercising**. Taking a drunk person on a brisk walk may seem like a good idea to sober them up, but it will not speed up the process of alcohol elimination, which occurs at a fixed rate in the liver.

Once a person has had too much to drink, they should be considered too impaired to function or drive until enough time has passed for the alcohol to be metabolized and removed from their system. While this may vary for each person, it generally takes someone with a 0.08 blood alcohol level approximately five hours to become completely sober.

ALCOHOLISM DEFINED

For most adults, drinking alcoholic beverages is a normal, harmless, even occasionally healthy activity. However, for some drinkers—1 in 13, according to the National Institute of Alcohol Abuse and Alcoholism—alcohol becomes a fixation that cannot be ignored or controlled. For those people, drinking is a disorder called alcoholism.

The term *alcoholism* describes a drinker who is physically and mentally dependent on alcohol, and who would likely suffer withdrawal symptoms upon quitting. This dependence prevents most alcoholics from being able to control when and how much they drink. For that reason, alcoholics usually drink excessively despite often devastating consequences, which can include problems with interpersonal relationships, deteriorating performance at school or work, impaired driving, and even brain damage. Alcoholism, like any addiction, involves continued use despite negative consequences. It is a chronic disorder requiring ongoing management and treatment.

THE IMPACT OF OVERUSE

Because many alcoholics don't report their condition or may not be aware of their dependence on alcohol, it is impossible to say exactly how many people suffer from alcoholism. However, some statistics paint a compelling picture of the effects of alcohol on society. According to the Centers for Disease Control and Prevention:

- About 79,000 deaths can be blamed on excessive alcohol use each year in the United States, which makes it the third-leading cause of lifestyle-related deaths.
- In 2005, more than 1.6 million hospitalizations and over 4 million emergency room visits were attributable to alcohol-related conditions.
- Alcohol use is a factor in two out of three instances of partner abuse.
- In 2005, almost 13,000 people died from alcohol-related liver disease.
- The National Survey on Drug Use and Health reported that in 2006 and 2007, about 2.2 million people in the United States attended a self-help group because of their alcohol use.
- The National Highway Transportation Safety Administration recorded 12,998 traffic fatalities caused by alcohol-related impairment—about a third of all traffic fatalities for the year.

Most instances of drinking, however, are not a sign of trouble. In some cultures, people begin drinking alcoholic beverages at an early age during meals or special ceremonies. For example:

- In the Catholic faith, adults and children alike may drink small amounts of wine during communion.
- For observant Jews, wine is a traditional part of the ritual celebration of Passover.
- In some Mediterranean countries like Italy and Greece, it's normal to serve wine and beer with meals, and teenagers are often permitted to drink these alcoholic beverages at an earlier age than their peers in other countries.

In most cultures, moderate drinking is a perfectly acceptable way to enjoy a meal, relax with friends, or celebrate a special occasion. There are some people, however, who should never drink, such as pregnant women, anyone planning on driving or operating heavy machinery, people taking certain medications that may interact dangerously with alcohol, people with liver disease, and anyone recovering from alcoholism or other addictions. Anyone with a family history of alcoholism may also want to approach drinking cautiously, even though not everyone with that genetic and environmental background is destined to become an alcoholic.

Fortunately, like many diseases, alcoholism can be treated, although it often takes lifelong commitment, support, and strong follow-through on the part of the drinker and his or her loved ones. As the research and medical communities have worked to develop an increasingly sophisticated understanding of alcoholism and addiction, in general, treatment options have advanced. Getting an alcoholic to admit to having a problem and then submit to screening tests, however, is still a common challenge.

ALCOHOLISM VS. ALCOHOL DEPENDENCY VS. ALCOHOL ABUSE

In addition to alcoholism, the terms *alcohol dependence* and *alcohol abuse* are also common. While abuse and dependence are often classified as two categories of alcoholism, many experts use the term *alcoholism* interchangeably with *alcohol dependence*. The latter leads to the former. However, to avoid the negative and ambiguous connotation of the word "alcoholism," many treatment professionals lean toward the more definable terms alcohol abuse and alcohol dependence.

The National Institute of Alcohol Abuse and Alcoholism characterizes alcohol abuse as a harmful form of drinking that leads to problems like disruptions in school or work, drunk driving, fighting, or becoming physically ill. People who abuse alcohol may continue to drink despite such mishaps, but they aren't physically addicted to alcohol and wouldn't experience physical withdrawal symptoms if they stopped.

Alcoholism arises from alcohol dependence, in which people feel a compulsion to drink and experience physical withdrawal symptoms if they don't drink. Alcoholics are plagued by the urge to drink, becoming preoccupied and scheduling other activities around drinking.

Why is this distinction important? By determining whether someone's behavior arises from alcohol abuse or dependence, clinicians and family members are more likely to find the most effective and targeted solution. For example, someone who abuses alcohol but isn't an alcoholic may want to join a self-help group to explore his or her reasons for drinking excessively—but that person may not necessarily need to take an anti-craving or other drug meant for someone with a more physically addictive drinking problem.

Are All Heavy Drinkers Alcoholics?

If someone drinks a lot, it can be hard to detect when he or she transitions from drinking heavily to abusing alcohol to being an actual alcoholic. Many people simply have a high tolerance for alcohol and may drink frequently without developing an addiction. Others may develop a dependence on alcohol after drinking only for a short time. Also, if someone is drinking heavily because of an underlying emotional or psychological issue, addressing the problem may cause the person to decrease or stop drinking with no problem. In the field of alcoholism treatment, there is no exact consensus on what types of drinkers correlate with which alcohol-related conditions, but a lot of overlap exists in professional definitions:

- American Medical Association (AMA) and American Society of Addiction Medicine (ASAM): A primary, chronic disease with genetic, psychosocial, and environmental factors influencing its development and manifestations. The disease is often progressive and fatal. It is characterized by impaired control over drinking, preoccupation with the drug alcohol, use of alcohol despite adverse consequences, and distortions in thinking, most notably denial. Each of these symptoms may be continuous or periodic.
- American Psychological Association (APA): People with alcoholism—technically known as alcohol dependence—have lost reliable control of their alcohol use. It doesn't matter what kind of alcohol someone drinks or even how much: alcohol-dependent people are often unable to stop drinking once they start. Alcohol dependence is characterized by tolerance (the need to drink more to achieve the same "high") and withdrawal symptoms if drinking is suddenly stopped.
- National Institute on Alcohol Abuse and Alcoholism (NIAAA): Alcoholism, also known as alcohol dependence, is a disease that includes the following four symptoms:
  - Craving—A strong need, or urge, to drink.
  - Loss of control—Not being able to stop drinking once drinking has begun.
  - Physical dependence—Withdrawal symptoms, such as nausea, sweating, shakiness, and anxiety after stopping drinking.
  - Tolerance—The need to drink greater amounts of alcohol to get "high."
- Alcoholics Anonymous (AA): An illness, a progressive illness, which can never be cured but, which, like some other diseases, can be arrested. The

illness represents the combination of a physical sensitivity to alcohol and a mental obsession with drinking, which, regardless of consequences, cannot be broken by willpower alone.

Some substance abuse professionals use the number of drinks per night or per week as a means of identifying someone who is at high risk for developing an alcohol use disorder. According to the Centers for Disease Control and Prevention, heavy drinking is defined as an average of more than 7 drinks per week for women and more than 14 drinks per week for men. Additionally, consuming more than 3 drinks in a night is considered a binge for a woman, with more than 4 drinks per night for a man. Anyone who regularly exceeds these limits for drinks per day and drinks per week is at high risk for developing alcoholism.

Among these varying definitions of alcoholism, all identify alcohol dependence as an illness, as opposed to moral failing or weakness of character. But healthcare professionals screen people for alcoholism differently than others. For a concerned layman, for example, the best way to determine if someone is an alcoholic may be simply to observe him or her for signs and symptoms of alcoholism. When a problem with alcohol is obvious, a commonsense approach can often confirm any doubt.

In observing someone who may have a drinking problem, it is important to remember that only a qualified clinician can make a formal diagnosis of alcoholism. However, once a concerned family member or friend has identified signs of alcohol dependence, this can serve as a first step toward a more clinical assessment. Plus, friends and family often see the alcoholic when he or she has been drinking, while clinicians usually don't have such an opportunity.

SIGNS AND SYMPTOMS

Most alcoholics won't admit to having a dependence on alcohol. This reluctance to disclose their condition can make it tricky to diagnose and treat them. Therefore, it's usually up to the people around them to know the signs of alcoholism, which include:

- Drinking alone
- Hiding how much and how often one drinks
- Becoming irritable or panicky during times when a drink is expected (such as before a meal)
- Needing more alcohol over time to feel its effects
- Problems at work, in relationships, or with money
- Needing to drink in order to relax or function normally
- Drinking with the intention of getting drunk
- Not enjoying pastimes or activities that were once considered fun

- Drinking to the point of "blacking out"—not remembering conversations or other activities that may have happened during a bout of drinking
- Showing signs of physical withdrawal after a period of not drinking, such as when waking up in the morning
- Losing interest in personal appearance
- Moodiness or personality changes, such as becoming hostile or violent after drinking
- Drinking early in the day
- Physiological signs and symptoms from long-term drinking, such as cirrhosis, ulcers, or memory loss.

Physical symptoms of alcoholism include:

- Abdominal pain
- Disorientation
- Being unable to stop drinking
- Nausea and vomiting
- Trembling (especially in the morning)
- Loss of appetite

Even the most heavily addicted drinker is unlikely to show every sign and symptom, and not every alcoholic will display the same ones. Some problem drinkers may only noticeably show one or two symptoms, and certain signs, like physical withdrawal symptoms, indicate particular trouble.

Withdrawal Symptoms

In some drinkers, the body develops a tolerance for alcohol and then can't function properly without it. This is known as withdrawal. Alcoholics suffering from physical withdrawal may have these symptoms:

- Uncontrollable shaking
- Anxiety
- Restlessness
- Appetite loss
- Vomiting or nausea
- Elevated blood pressure, heart rate, or temperature
- Seizures
- Confusion
- Profuse sweating
- Delirium tremens

One of the most ferocious forms of alcohol withdrawal is delirium tremens, or DTs. This condition arises from the effect of heavy drinking on a neurotransmitter in the brain called gamma-aminobutyric acid, or GABA.

GABA is critical for calming the excitable neurotransmitters of the brain (such as epinephrine), providing a balance to maintain a proper sleep cycle, keep anxiety in check, and, if necessary, prevent seizures. Alcohol stimulates the brain's GABA receptors, exerting a calming effect, which explains how drinking can make people relax or lose their inhibitions.

When some alcoholics stop drinking, their GABA levels decrease, causing an increase in the more stimulating neurotransmitters that are normally balanced out by GABA. This can cause existing symptoms of alcohol withdrawal to progress to DTs. Symptoms of DTs are severe and may include:

- Delirium (waxing and waning of consciousness)
- Delusions (beliefs or thoughts that contradict reality)
- Hallucinations
- High fever
- Confusion
- Profuse sweating
- Psychotic behavior, including hallucinations
- Insomnia
- Seizures
- Extreme agitation
- Panic attacks
- Paranoia
- Racing pulse

DTs is considered a medical emergency that can be fatal, but if it is treated right away, the symptoms are usually temporary and disappear after a few days, leaving the person weakened but able to recover with medical care and other forms of support. Only a small percentage of alcoholics in withdrawal experience DTs. If not treated in a medical setting, DTs can be fatal in about one-third of cases. Treated in a medical facility, the fatality rate is much lower, around 3 percent.

What to Look For

Perhaps the most compelling evidence of alcohol dependence is when the drinker makes alcohol a priority over all other activities or pastimes. For example, it may be noticed that the alcoholic finds drinking more important than relationships or work performance. Or the person may schedule social engagements, vacations, or other activities around drinking, making sure alcohol is always part of the plan.

This compulsion to put alcohol at the center of everything is at the root of all other symptoms of alcoholism. For example, if someone chooses to drink even though the smell of alcohol on the breath would jeopardize his or her job, this is a clear sign that the prospect of drinking far outweighs the risk of being fired.

CAUSES OF ALCOHOLISM

While many theories exist on the causes of alcoholism, one thing most researchers and drinkers agree on is that the addiction doesn't happen all at once. This is a disease that takes hold of a person slowly, over time. The causes are multifaceted and complex, becoming better understood with each decade of substance abuse research.

In looking at the causes of alcoholism, two issues should be considered: the reasons people drink, and the reasons a certain percentage of those people become dependent on alcohol. For example, if someone started drinking heavily to cope with the loss of a spouse, he or she may seek counseling, recover from the worst of the grief, and then be able cut down on drinking with no withdrawal symptoms. Someone else in a similar situation may also be able to resolve their grief, but then find that they have developed a dependence on alcohol and can no longer cut down without help. In identifying some common causes for alcohol dependence, substance abuse experts and clinicians have also been able to identify people at risk for alcoholism.

Why Some People Become Addicted

There are many reasons why people drink. But when does normal alcohol consumption turn into addiction? Why can some people drink excessively but stop with no physical problems, while others become dependent on alcohol? According to the National Institutes of Health (NIH), the most likely causes for alcohol addiction are genetics, environment, and neurology.

Genetics

The fact that alcoholism sometimes runs in families led to the theory that there is a genetic component to this and other addictions. In fact, scientists have already gathered enough evidence to support the idea of a genetically inherited predisposition to alcoholism.

Genetic factors can occur in many parts of the body affected by alcohol. For example, there may be a variation that affects how the liver breaks alcohol down, which would affect how quickly someone would feel the intoxicating effects of drinking, as well as what their specific reaction would be. Another variation may present itself as a booster for the receptors of certain neurotransmitters affected by drinking, which could increase a person's vulnerability to the alcohol addiction. And yet a third variation presents itself as differences in opiate receptors, which can vary even from alcoholic to alcoholic, and which can make an individual more prone to alcoholism.

This doesn't mean that every alcoholic was born with a genetic predisposition that explains away the problem, nor does it mean that anyone with certain genetic markers for alcoholism will develop a problem. It does indicate, however, that some people are more susceptible than others to become physically dependent on alcohol. But genetics is only one factor in alcohol dependence. As stated by the National Institute on Alcohol Abuse and Alcoholism in its July 2003 issue of *Alcohol Alert*:

> Like diabetes and heart disease, alcoholism is considered genetically complex, distinguishing it from genetic diseases, such as cystic fibrosis, that result primarily from the action of one or two copies of a single gene and in which the environment plus a much smaller role, if any.
>
> In addition to the genes a person inherits from his or her parents, factors like culture and upbringing may also determine the likelihood of developing alcoholism.

Environment

Kids in certain home or social environments may be more likely to develop a problem with alcohol later in life. For example, according to the American Academy of Child & Adolescent Psychiatry, children of alcoholics are four times more likely to become alcoholics themselves. But not every child in such an environment will develop a drinking problem.

Underage drinkers may also be influenced by other factors in their environment, such as availability and cost of alcohol, friends' use of alcohol, advertising, and the portrayal of drinking in movies and television. Adults are also susceptible to environmental factors, including social situations, pressures at work or at home, their friends, and how much their spouse or partner drinks.

Neurology

Over time, drinking disrupts the normal balance of the brain's neurotransmitters, and some people may find they need to drink to feel "right." To compensate for changes in neurotransmitter activity due to drinking, the brain may signal the body to start craving alcohol to keep chemicals in balance. As this happens, alcohol use can gradually turn into alcohol addiction, as the brain loses the ability altogether to establish this balance on its own.

WHO IS AT RISK?

There is no way to identify a single cause for any individual's dependence on alcohol. For example, if someone's family history includes ample alcohol dependence, that person's risk of becoming an alcoholic could be equally attributable to both genetics and environment. But the person is clearly at risk. Aside from genetics and family history, other risk factors include:

- Prolonged periods of steady or heavy drinking (defined by the National Institute on Alcohol Abuse and Alcoholism as more than 14 drinks weekly for men, or more than 7 drinks weekly for women).
- Trauma, such as witnessing an act of violence, experiencing a car accident, or being in an abusive relationship.
- Underage drinking. According to the Centers for Disease Control and Prevention, young people who start drinking before age 15 are five times more likely to become alcohol abusers or alcoholics as adults than their peers who don't start drinking until age 21.
- Being a male. The National Institute on Alcohol Abuse and Alcoholism reports that men are more likely than women to become alcoholics, perhaps because they can metabolize alcohol more readily and therefore are less apt to feel its unpleasant effects as quickly.
- Mood disorders. According to the American Psychiatric Association, people suffering from depression or anxiety are more vulnerable to alcohol addiction.
- Race. Due to certain genetic differences in alcohol-metabolizing enzymes among people of different races, some ethnic populations are more susceptible to addiction. For example, Native Americans seem to be more at risk for alcoholism than African Americans and Asian Americans are. Additionally, Asian Americans lack a key enzyme needed to metabolize alcohol, so they suffer unpleasant effects from drinking, such as facial flushing, that decrease their odds of developing a tolerance to alcohol.

HEALTH COMPLICATIONS

Virtually every system in the body is adversely affected by heavy or long-term drinking, from the heart to the brain to the skin (see Figure 2.1). Although the body can adjust to the effects of moderate drinking, once a person exceeds the acceptable amount of alcohol, any manner of physical or neurological damage can result. Health problems may not even be limited to the drinker, as in the case of pregnant women who make the unfortunate decision to use alcohol.

The following organs and body systems are most affected by long-term excessive use of alcohol:

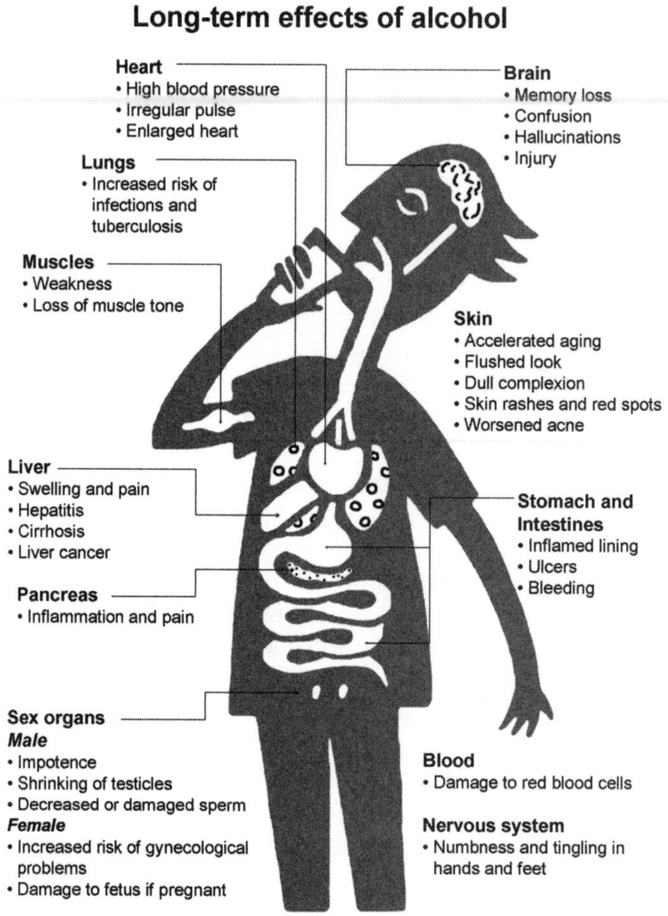

Long-term effects of alcohol

Heart
• High blood pressure
• Irregular pulse
• Enlarged heart

Lungs
• Increased risk of
  infections and
  tuberculosis

Muscles
• Weakness
• Loss of muscle tone

Liver
• Swelling and pain
• Hepatitis
• Cirrhosis
• Liver cancer

Pancreas
• Inflammation and pain

Sex organs
Male
• Impotence
• Shrinking of testicles
• Decreased or damaged sperm
Female
• Increased risk of gynecological
  problems
• Damage to fetus if pregnant

Brain
• Memory loss
• Confusion
• Hallucinations
• Injury

Skin
• Accelerated aging
• Flushed look
• Dull complexion
• Skin rashes and red spots
• Worsened acne

**Stomach and
Intestines**
• Inflamed lining
• Ulcers
• Bleeding

Blood
• Damage to red blood cells

Nervous system
• Numbness and tingling in
  hands and feet

Figure 2.1 Long-term, excessive use of alcohol can cause many adverse physical effects and damage every organ and system in the body. [Illustrator: G. Brennan]

Liver

Of all the health issues associated with drinking, liver problems probably come to mind first. The liver can break down and metabolize alcohol at the rate of about one drink per hour, so it is easy to see why consistently flooding it with more alcohol could interfere with its ability to do its job. Heavy or prolonged drinking can lead to serious liver-related illnesses, including:

• Alcoholic hepatitis (not to be confused with infectious forms of hepatitis, like hepatitis B), an inflammation of the liver that predisposes someone for cirrhosis. Symptoms include fever, abdominal pain, and yellowing of the skin and eyes (jaundice).

- Cirrhosis, an irreversible destruction and scarring of the liver (see Figure 2.2). This condition appears in about 20 percent of people with alcoholic hepatitis. Its effects can be life-threatening, especially in people who continue to drink after being diagnosed. Because of the liver's critical role in many essential life processes, damage caused by cirrhosis can have widespread secondary effects, including:
    - Vitamin deficiency. Because alcohol interferes with the liver's ability to store calcium and fat-soluble vitamins (A, D, E, and K), heavy drinking over time can lead to vitamin deficiencies, triggering secondary issues such as vision problems.
    - Decreased fat absorption. Because fat is where calcium is stored, when the liver can no longer absorb fat in sufficient amounts, bones may become thinner or more brittle from lack of calcium.
    - Cell structure damage from protein deficiency, because heavy drinking causes the liver to produce less protein.
    - Portal hypertension, a dangerous type of high blood pressure that occurs when blood can no longer move freely through the scarred tissue of an alcohol-damaged liver.
    - Ascites, a pooling of tissue fluid that the liver deposits into the abdominal cavity because it can no longer transport it to the circulatory system. The most common symptom is a distended (protruding) belly.
    - Low blood sugar due to the liver's diminished ability to extract glucose from food.
    - Low glycogen stores. A cirrhotic liver can't store glycogen as well as it normally does, which means less usable sugar available to power energy-intensive cellular work.

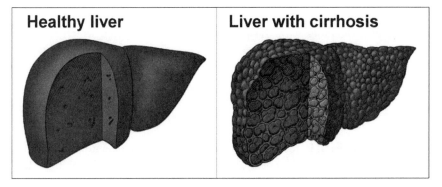

Figure 2.2 Years of heavy drinking can cause a healthy liver (left) to develop cirrhosis (right), a disease that destroys and scars liver tissue and can interfere with normal liver functioning, often resulting in irreversible liver damage. [Mayo Foundation for Medical Education and Research, all rights reserved]

Digestive System

In the pancreas, excessive alcohol use can decrease digestive enzymes sent to the stomach, which impairs digestion. In the stomach, damage from heavy drinking can damage the stomach walls, leading to diminished absorption, decreased protein formation, and gastrointestinal bleeding.

Blood

Since drinking reduces the ability of bone marrow to use iron to make hemoglobin, it may be a culprit in some forms of anemia (insufficient red blood cells, or RBCs). Also, gastrointestinal bleeding caused by dammage to the stomach from heavy drinking may lead to anemia.

Heavy drinking cuts the already brief lifespan of an RBC in half, often because the spleen is damaged and unable to distinguish good RBCs from damaged ones, destroying both types in the process. And RBCs affected by alcohol may also clump together, presenting circulation problems and increasing the possibility of blood clots.

White blood cells (WBCs) may also become damaged by excessive drinking, which reduces the body's ability to fight infections. In addiction, excess alcohol impairs the immune system's killer white cells, an important component in preventing cancer. Furthermore, alcohol may prevent otherwise healthy WBCs from sticking to and eliminating harmful bacteria.

Finally, many heavy drinkers may develop problems with platelet formation. Platelets are critical for wound healing, causing blood to clot to prevent further bleeding. As a result, some alcoholics develop bruises easily.

Endocrine System

In addition to the digestive problems related to an alcohol-impaired pancreas, drinking also interferes with the pancreas's insulin secretion, which makes it harder for the body to regulate blood sugar levels. This is particularly dangerous for people with diabetes who drink excessively and may already be having blood sugar problems.

Cardiovascular System

Although research in recent decades has shown that moderate drinking may have beneficial effects on the heart, this doesn't apply to heavy drinking. Alcohol-related risks to the cardiovascular system include:

- High blood pressure, which increases the likelihood of heart attack or stroke.

- Coronary artery disease, due to elevated levels of cholesterol and triglycerides, substances that, in high amounts, can block arteries and impair circulation.
- Myocarditis, an inflammation of the heart muscle, caused by alcohol-related toxicity that makes it harder for the heart to get the proper amount of blood to the rest of the body. This can lead to congestive heart failure and fluid buildup in the lungs, among other problems.
- Alcoholic cardiomyopathy, a condition that weakens and inflames the heart muscle, impairing its ability to pump blood with enough pressure to reach the outermost blood vessels of the body, such as those in the feet and hands.
- Increased heart rate or arrhythmia (irregular heartbeat), which puts increased strain on the heart muscle. A rapid pulse caused by a condition called sinus tachycardia may also occur as a result of alcohol's effect on stress hormones.

Brain

The main factor influencing alcohol's effect on the brain appears to be blood alcohol level, particularly when the level is increasing rather than decreasing. In nonalcoholics, the blood alcohol concentration needed to trigger signs of drunkenness is lower than full-fledged heavy drinkers, whose high tolerance may camouflage the devastating effects of alcohol on the brain. In addition to alcohol's effects on the brain's neurotransmitters, other problems may arise from heavy drinking, including:

- **Wernicke-Korsakoff syndrome**. This brain disease is sometimes separated into two conditions: Wernicke's encephalopathy and Korsakoff's dementia (or Korsakoff's psychosis). The disorder arises from the thiamine deficiency that can result from alcohol's toxic effect on the body's absorption abilities. It's often considered a form of dementia, with similar symptoms such as delirium, fearfulness, confusion, and problems with walking. Rather than causing the memory loss of, say, a blackout (an incident of amnesia, or inability to remember past events), Wernicke-Korsakoff syndrome inhibits the individual's ability to form new memories (anterograde amnesia). This can lead to creating events that never occurred to fill in memory gaps caused by drinking (confabulation).
- **Amnesia**. At certain blood alcohol levels (0.20 or higher), some drinkers may experience memory problems or black out altogether. A blackout is a form of alcohol-related amnesia, where the person may appear to be conscious and functioning fairly normally, but then may not remember events or conversations later.
- **Dementia**. Heavy drinking can increase the incidences of small undetectable strokes that damage the brain slowly over time, leading to a condition known

as vascular dementia. Symptoms include confusion, agitation, unsteady movement, urinary problems, and mood swings. This is not the same kind of dementia caused by Wernicke-Krosakoff syndrome.

- **Abstinence syndrome.** If someone drinks regularly and excessively over time, the brain makes adjustments to accommodate the neurological effects of the alcohol. Eventually this adaptation turns into physical dependence and the body will experience withdrawal symptoms if the person doesn't drink. Abstinence syndrome refers to the physiological effects of this dependence, which are the opposite of the effects of drinking. Symptoms include trembling, sleeplessness, hallucinations, anxiousness, restlessness, and irritability.

Lungs

The effect of drinking on lung health is a relatively new field of study, although alcohol has long been identified as a risk factor for lung infections such as pneumonia and tuberculosis. New research shows that prolonged alcohol use may cause lung scarring that resembles that of cirrhosis of the liver.

A 2008 report from the journal *Alcohol Research and Health* highlighted a study group of people at risk for developing acute respiratory distress syndrome (ARDS), an inflammatory lung disease that causes shortness of breath and other symptoms. In the study, alcoholics were 21 percent more likely to acquire ARDS than their nondrinking peers with other ARDS risk factors.

Sexual Problems

How alcohol affects sexual behavior is complex. On one hand, by lowering inhibitions, drinking can make a person more sexually active than they would be otherwise. While this might not be a bad thing in and of itself, it can lead to unprotected sex, which increases the risks of unwanted pregnancy and sexually transmitted diseases. On the other hand, excessive drinking can make it harder to have and enjoy sex, often causing problems with male sexual performance. By elevating blood pressure and cholesterol levels, alcohol can cause impotence. Circulatory problems can cause vascular problems that lead to erectile dysfunction.

People whose drinking leads to a condition called peripheral neuropathy— nerve damage to the hands, legs, and feet that can cause numbness, tingling, and weakness—may have difficulties feeling sexual pleasure due to the diminished nerve supply to the genitals.

Pregnancy and the Female Reproductive System

A woman who drinks while pregnant puts the fetus at risk for a set of symptoms known as fetal alcohol syndrome (FAS). Possible birth defects from drinking during pregnancy range from mild cognitive problems to severe developmental disabilities that require lifelong care. According to the National Institute on Alcohol Abuse and Alcoholism, Fetal Alcohol Syndrome is the leading known preventable cause of mental retardation. Effects of FAS may include:

- Abnormal facial development
- Retarded growth
- Brain damage that can lead to impaired intelligence and behavioral problems
- Learning disabilities, especially around language and spatial relationships
- Attention disorders similar to attention-deficit/hyperactivity disorder
- Diminished brain functions, such as problem-solving, abstract thinking, planning, and organizing
- Low birth weight
- Smaller head size

A woman does not need to be an alcoholic for drinking to put her baby at risk for FAS—any amount of drinking can be dangerous during pregnancy. And drinking during pregnancy may not always lead to actual FAS. A less severe range of alcohol-related problems, known as fetal alcohol effects (FAE), may trigger milder abnormalities. Even before a woman becomes pregnant, she may experience alcohol-related problems in the reproductive system, including erratic periods and decreased fertility.

Interactions with Medications

People who drink while taking certain medications, prescription or otherwise, run the risk of unpleasant or even dangerous side effects. This is generally simple to avoid since most drugs and medicines are clearly labeled to warn against such interactions. Heavy drinkers who avoid such warnings could put themselves in danger, depending on the drug and amount of alcohol consumed. In fact, in some years, such interactions alone are a factor in 1 out of 4 emergency room admissions, according to the National Institute on Alcohol Abuse and Alcoholism.

In some cases, the body uses the same mechanisms to metabolize and eliminate alcohol that it uses for medications. If certain digestive enzymes are being taken up by alcohol, the medication may take longer to exit the body because it has to wait its turn to be metabolized. In this waiting state, the drug may stay in the body longer, increasing the chances for overdose or side effects. In other cases, alcohol simply reduces the effectiveness of certain medications, which can be catastrophic for people relying on life-saving medications, such as antiseizure drugs.

Symptoms of such interactions vary in type and severity, depending on the drug being used, the amount of alcohol consumed, the person's age and health, and other factors. Common symptoms include sleepiness, fainting, stumbling, nausea, vomiting, and dizziness. Even more dangerous are side effects such as gastric bleeding, shortness of breath, and rapid heartbeat. Some interactions may even make the medication harmful to the body.

The easiest way to avoid such interactions is to pay close attention to warning labels regarding alcohol and medications. Even certain nonprescription (over-the-counter) medications or herbal supplements can be harmful if taken with alcohol. Members of populations that tend to take more prescription medications, such as older people, are more at risk for reactions.

Social Complications of Drinking

In addition to the physical effects of alcoholism, there are psychological and social complications to consider, including:

- **Drunk driving**. Alcohol affects the parts of the brain that control the functions that are most important for driving safely: reaction time, clear-headedness, assessing danger, and multitasking. Alcohol-related accidents account for a third of all traffic fatalities, making drunk driving one of the most preventable causes of death in the United States.
- **Impaired performance at work and at school**. Over time, alcohol's effect on the brain inevitably compromises even the most accomplished student's or employee's efforts to perform at their best.
- **Relationship problems**. When one person in a relationship (whether it is a marriage, friendship, or parent–child relationship) becomes so dependent on alcohol that drinking becomes the central priority, the relationship is often destined for rocky times. People suffering from alcoholism often hide their addiction and may use drinking as a way to avoid communicating with their partners, friends, parents, or other loved ones.

Health Benefits for the Moderate Drinker

Moderate drinking may show some benefits for the heart. In 2003, the *New England Journal of Medicine* published an article by a team of researchers who discovered lower rates of heart attack among men who drank several times a week compared to men who didn't. Other studies have shown alcohol's beneficial effects in lowering blood cholesterol levels, which in turn reduces the risk of coronary artery disease. This has been particularly true in cultures that drink a lot of wine, leading researchers to dub this the "French Paradox." Scientists are still trying to determine the beneficial properties of wine and how they work, so this phenomenon is still not fully understood.

In the last decade, many studies like these have surfaced. The findings have triggered much attention and with good reason. Drinking is a pleasurable activity for many people, so the idea of alcohol also providing health benefits is an irresistible thought. But it is important to look closely at these preliminary results, with the main idea being moderation. No study is ever likely to unearth any benefits from the heavy drinking associated with alcoholism.

MORAL FAILING OR LEGITIMATE DISEASE?

People who are not alcoholics may have a hard time understanding how a seemingly voluntary behavior like drinking can be labeled as an illness or disease. This is understandable, because most of us think of a disease as something a person has no control over. Alcohol is not infectious, like measles or pneumonia. It is not spontaneous and involuntary, like cancer or diabetes, where something measurable or visible has gone wrong. It is not caused by an insect bite, virus, bacteria, or airborne germ. It does not show up on an X-ray. So what makes it a disease?

To understand why alcoholism is a disease, it is important to know about the neurological effects of alcohol on the brain. Simply put, heavy drinking over time causes changes in neurotransmitter activity that the brain must adapt to. In people physically predisposed to alcoholism, this adaptation eventually turns into a fixed craving as the body finds it cannot live without the effects of alcohol. Something that started out voluntary and enjoyable turns into something more serious—a physical dependence that can cause horrible withdrawal symptoms. This explains why alcoholics cannot just quit drinking like their nonaddicted counterparts can.

Thus, it is not the behavior of drinking that is defined as an illness. It is only when the craving to drink becomes involuntary that alcoholism can be thought of as a disease. This loss of control over drinking may be attributable to genetics, psychological factors, the environment, or a combination of any of these.

Agreeing to Disagree

Despite efforts to classify alcoholism as a disease, however, not all scientists, clinicians, and academic researchers agree that the compulsion to drink belongs

---

What Doctors Really Think

Although the official clinical position is that alcohol is a disease, many doctors disagree. A 1997 survey among physicians showed that 80 percent of those questioned believe that alcoholism is a personal conduct problem rather than a disease, an attitude that may influence a physician's approach to alcoholism diagnosis and treatment.

in the category of illness. Some critics of the idea see this as absolving drinkers of any responsibility for their condition and classify alcoholism as an extension of a drinking-centric lifestyle. Others think the disease theory of alcoholism means alcoholics will seek out a physician-mediated cure, such as a medication or procedure, with both patient and doctor neglecting the more complex reasons for drinking. Where the two camps may come together, however, is in expanding the definition of disease to include nonpathological factors like societal influences and environment (such as home life), which may apply to other diseases as well (such as depression).

It may also be easier to think of alcoholism as a chronic illness, with the same hallmarks of all chronic illnesses—a gradual onset, symptoms that flare-up and then ebb again, identifying lifestyle changes needed to prevent flare-ups, and the need for emotional support from family and friends. Compare alcoholism with diabetes, for example, where people have tools and resources at their disposal to manage a voluntary behavior (i.e., unhealthy eating) that, if not controlled, could lead to serious health problems.

Because of the physically addictive nature of alcohol, most alcoholics are unable or unlikely to quit on their own. In fact, just admitting to an addiction is enough of a challenge for most alcoholics, and sometimes an intervention by family and friends is the only way to get a drinker to agree to a recovery program. Denial of any problem with alcohol, combined with reluctance to give up something their body craves so fiercely, can dampen the prospect for quitting permanently without help. For most alcoholics, the chances for successfully giving up drinking are much higher with treatment and support from loved ones.

3

Diagnosing and
Treating Alcoholism

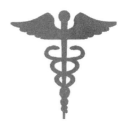

Alcoholism is a chronic disease, one that requires serious intervention followed by a lifelong commitment to prevent relapse and establish permanent abstinence. A variety of resources are available to help alcoholics identify their level of dependence, receive screening tests and evaluation, explore their reasons for drinking, and work with doctors, nurses, counselors, and other clinicians to find a treatment program that best fits their needs. Like any other chronic illnesses, alcoholism should be thought of as a treatable condition.

ALCOHOLISM: CHRONIC AND COMPLICATED

With many chronic illnesses, such as diabetes or depression, a person may notice symptoms early enough to get treatment before the disease progresses. However, the addictive nature of alcoholism prevents many drinkers from seeking or even accepting treatment until the illness has reached a crisis point, whether it is physical signs of withdrawal, personal problems, or a serious health problem. For this reason, treating alcoholism can be more complicated than treating other chronic illnesses. Determining a diagnosis of alcoholism alone involves choosing the correct screening tools and knowing which signs and symptoms to look for.

Making Sense of the Signs and Symptoms

Nothing about treating alcoholism is exact or precise. To determine whether someone has a drinking problem, family, friends, coworkers, and even clinicians are often confronted with a bewildering array of signs and symptoms, which may or may not provide clarity.

Some signs of alcoholism are obvious. For example, a person who shakes violently in the morning before having a drink is probably physically dependent. Blacking out is another sure sign of a drinking problem. But what about symptoms like drinking to get drunk? Could this simply be a sign of someone coping with stress instead of a sign of alcoholism? Similarly, moodiness and loss of appetite could be signs of an underlying problem camouflaged or accompanied by alcohol abuse.

The purpose of paying attention to the signs and symptoms of a problem drinker is not to make a diagnosis. Noting such behaviors or physical effects is useful for other reasons. For one thing, it's a good way for concerned family and friends to document the signs in order to start building a picture of the drinker's behavior. It may be startling to know how much tolerance a drinker has built up to alcohol, for example. Or maybe a person never noticed how moody the drinker becomes in the absence of alcohol.

Such observations, noted by people closest to the drinker, form a valuable body of knowledge for the clinician trying to make a formal diagnosis. The person most qualified to diagnose alcoholism doesn't usually get the chance to see the drinker on a day-to-day basis, least of all when the person is drinking heavily or drunk. Without this intimate view of the drinker, the clinician depends on others for insights about the person's drinking behavior.

That doesn't mean, however, that the person making the diagnosis cannot turn to other means for gathering information. Aside from signs and symptoms that may be present, clinicians can gather information from drinkers themselves, choosing from a variety of screening tools available.

SCREENING AND DIAGNOSIS

In determining whether someone has a problem with alcohol, the first step is often a screening test, which physicians, therapists, and other healthcare providers use in a variety of settings, from the doctor's office to the emergency room. The purpose of a screening test isn't to make a definitive diagnosis, but rather to determine the likelihood that someone may have a problem with alcohol and need to undergo diagnostic testing.

Most people, alcoholics and otherwise, have probably run across some form of screening test at some point in their lives, such as in a magazine article about alcohol consumption. These tests usually take the form of a questionnaire that inquires about frequency of drinking or amount of alcohol consumed. They're easy to administer and can often be completed by the drinker on his or her own. The most well-known types of available screening tests range in length from 1 to 25 questions. Each is designed to be used for different people or needs, including:

- Certain populations, such as minorities, students, or pregnant women
- Different settings (some work better in a doctor's office, while some may be given by a therapist)
- Type of drinking behavior (such as binge drinking)
- Type of drinking problem (alcohol abuser vs. alcoholic, for example)
- Amount of alcohol consumed—For example, if someone exceeds the U.S. government-indicated safety limit for drinks per day (one for women, two for men), it could indicate increased tolerance and eventual dependence.

Abuse or Dependence?

People with alcohol dependence are physically addicted to alcohol and would suffer physical withdrawal symptoms if they stopped drinking. Alcohol abusers may drink chronically and get themselves into trouble with alcohol-related incidents, but could stop without suffering physical effects. But that doesn't mean that alcohol abusers don't need treatment to help cope with underlying reasons for drinking and to prevent progressing to alcoholism. It's a risky assumption to consider alcohol abusers as less "in trouble" than people who are fully dependent on alcohol.

As an analogy, consider someone newly diagnosed with a precancerous skin growth that can often progress to skin cancer. That person wouldn't necessarily need the same intensive treatment as a person who already has skin cancer, but he or she would still be advised to see a dermatologist to have the growths examined and possibly removed, and to use sunblock and avoid the sun.

A person with a predependent form of alcohol use would likely be advised in the same way—to start receiving treatment before things get worse. Treatments for all types of problem drinkers may overlap. Brief intervention, counseling, and behavioral therapy may be the focus for alcohol abusers, with the addition of medication or inpatient treatment for actual alcoholics. Additionally, an accurate diagnosis can prevent alcohol abusers from being overdiagnosed with a more dependent form of alcohol behavior and from being prescribed medications or rehabilitation they don't need.

Today, substance abuse is thought of as a spectrum, with each level of use requiring different treatment approaches, and professionals who treat problem drinkers must make more careful assessments. Fortunately, many screening tools exist to help doctors and therapists make an accurate diagnosis.

Screening Tools for Alcohol Problems

There are several screening tests available to identify problem drinking and alcohol dependence. Choosing the best screening test is a key challenge for many substance abuse treatment professionals, who may have different criteria depending on the person being tested. A busy emergency room doctor would likely choose a brief questionnaire to assess someone quickly, while a therapist in a less urgent setting could choose a more extensive test to obtain a clearer picture of the person's drinking behavior.

In his book *Treating Alcohol Problems*, Dr. Frederick Rotgers identified these criteria for choosing an appropriate screening test:

- Brief and easy to administer
- Low cost and easy to obtain and score
- Written in nontechnical language
- Easy to interpret and explain
- Reliable and good at predicting real-world outcomes
- Sensitive to change

It's important to work with a practitioner who has experience and expertise in administering, scoring, and interpreting results. Some of the most commonly used screening tools for detecting alcohol problems are:

AUDIT

In 1982, the World Health Organization (WHO) developed the Alcohol Use Disorders Identification Test (AUDIT) screening test. WHO designed the AUDIT as a simple method of screening for excessive drinking and to assist in providing a brief assessment. It has become the standard screening test for many primary care providers, used more than others because of its accuracy in measuring a range of risky drinking behaviors, from the occasional binge drinker to the advanced alcoholic. AUDIT is also useful because it is appropriate for a wide variety of groups, such as hospital patients, people with mood disorders, inmates, homeless people who drink, and drunk drivers. Because the AUDIT is easy to use and administer, it is a useful screening tool in areas with limited healthcare practitioners and facilities. The test sets the stage for intervention, helping problem drinkers see the possible harmful outcomes of their addiction so they can take preventative steps.

AUDIT is used internationally, and in the last two decades its popularity has grown in parallel with the increasing use of alcohol screening. WHO has occasionally revised AUDIT to keep up with periodic advances in alcoholism screening research. The full-length AUDIT test features 10 questions:

- The first three questions measure how much a person drinks.
- Questions 4–6 are designed to detect possible symptoms of dependence.
- Questions 7–10 help identify the impact of drinking on everyday life.

Shorter versions are available for busier healthcare environments. One such version is the Fast Alcohol Screening Test (FAST), which extracts questions 3, 5, 8, and 10 from the AUDIT to help form a quicker assessment of alcohol-related behavior.

CAGE

The CAGE questionnaire is another popular assessment tool. It's short and simple, making it a less complicated choice for care providers than the AUDIT tool. It's also considered more accurate for detecting alcohol dependence rather than alcohol abuse, as well as alcohol use over a lifetime. The letters in CAGE serve as a memory tool for key words in the four questions asked:

- Have you ever felt you should Cut down on your drinking?
- Have people Annoyed you by criticizing your drinking?
- Have you ever felt bad or Guilty about your drinking?
- Have you ever had a drink first thing in the morning, an Eye opener, to steady your nerves or get rid of a hangover?

Answering "yes" to two or more questions is considered a positive result, suggestive of follow-up assessment.

Michigan Alcohol Screening Test

Another useful screening tool is the Michigan Alcohol Screening Test (MAST), developed in the 1970s as a 25-question assessment that has since been reduced to 22 questions. Its emphasis on long-term drinking patterns makes it especially helpful for identifying alcohol dependency, such as weekend binge drinking.

Like the AUDIT, the MAST has shorter versions, including the 10-question Brief MAST (BMAST) and the 13-question Short MAST. MAST also is versatile, being suitable for adults or adolescents, and easy to administer by either a clinician or layperson.

Quantity/Frequency Questionnaire

For situations that require a less time-consuming assessment than standard screening tools, the National Institute on Alcohol Abuse and Alcoholism developed the Quantity/Frequency Questionnaire. This short test contains three questions:

1. How many days per week do you drink alcohol on average?
2. How many drinks do you have on a typical day?
3. What is the maximum number of drink you've consumed on a single occasion in the past month?

If the answers to these questions reveal that the person's quantity and frequency of drinking exceeds standard limits of safe drinking, the test is considered positive. These results can be used as a basis for lengthier screening later.

Screening Tests for Women

Accurate screening tests for women have become a priority among substance abuse care providers and obstetricians alike, mainly because of the risk of alcohol's effects on a developing fetus. Dr. Grace Chang, an NIAAA researcher, identified several potential shortfalls in using traditional screening tests for female drinkers:

- The traditional screening tests were designed with men in mind. Men have different drinking patterns and behaviors than women and can withstand higher levels of alcohol before suffering health effects.
- Several of the tests were designed to detect alcohol dependence. This is not common in pregnant women, who nonetheless may be drinking enough to harm their babies.
- Pregnant women are more likely to deny or minimize their drinking due to shame and embarrassment.
- Most traditional screening tests include designated limits for safe drinking (such as having up to 2 drinks per day for men). For pregnant women, no universally safe level of drinking has been established.

There are two common alcohol screening tools designed for women:

TWEAK

This 5-question test can be used for both men and women, but has been shown to yield more accurate assessment results in pregnant women. It uses similar questions from other traditional screening tests:

- Tolerance (2 points): How many drinks can you hold? (Six or more indicates tolerance.)
- Worried (2 points): Have close friends or relatives worried or complained about your drinking in the past year?

- Eye openers (1 point): Do you sometimes take a drink in the morning when you first get up?
- Amnesia (1 point): Has a friend or family member ever told you about things you said or did while you were drinking that you could not remember?
- K(C)ut down (1 point): Do you sometimes feel the need to cut down on your drinking?

On a 7-point scale, women taking the TWEAK test are considered at-risk drinkers if they score 2 or more points.

T-ACE

This 4-question assessment is based on CAGE and is useful for detecting how much a woman may be drinking during pregnancy, as well as alcohol consumed before pregnancy (an often overlooked pregnancy risk factor) and lifetime drinking patterns:

- Tolerance: How many drinks does it take to make you feel high? (2 points for 2 or more drinks per day)
- Have people Annoyed you by criticizing your drinking? (1 point if yes)
- Have you ever felt you had to Cut down on your drinking? (1 point if yes)
- Have you ever had a drink first thing in the morning (Eye opener) to steady your nerves or get rid of a hangover? (1 point if yes)

A score of 2 or higher is considered a positive outcome for pregnancy risk drinking.

CRAFFT

Most screening tests were designed with adult drinkers in mind and may not take into account the factors that can cause teens to drink, such as the need to fit in. The CRAFFT screening tool was designed by the Center for Adolescent Substance Abuse Research at Children's Hospital Boston to help pediatricians and other healthcare providers detect substance abuse in young people. The CRAFFT test consists of a short list of six questions:

- Have you ever ridden in a Car driven by someone (including yourself) who was "high" or had been using alcohol or drugs?
- Do you ever use alcohol or drugs to Relax, feel better about yourself, or fit in?
- Do you ever use alcohol/drugs while you are by yourself, Alone?
- Do you ever Forget things you did while using alcohol or drugs?

- Do your family or Friends ever tell you that you should cut down on your drinking or drug use?
- Have you gotten into Trouble while you were using alcohol or drugs?

Two or more "Yes" answers indicate a serious problem.

Lab Tests for Alcoholism

While there is no test that can provide a definitive diagnosis of alcoholism, certain laboratory tests can indicate heavy or prolonged drinking:

- Blood alcohol level through breath analysis—a common indicator of very recent drinking (used most often to detect drunk driving), but not useful for determining much else (such as how long the person has been drinking).
- Liver enzyme tests—since the liver is the organ that sustains the most damage from drinking, someone who drinks a lot is likely to show elevated levels of certain liver enzymes, such as gamma-glutyl transpeptidase (GGT).
- Mean corpuscular volume (MCV)—low values for this can reveal an alcohol-triggered vitamin deficiency that has led to macrocytic anemia.
- Low platelet count—due to alcohol's damage to factors involved in the clotting process.
- Carbohydrate-deficient transferrin (CDT)—high values for this blood test indicate recent, prolonged, and heavy alcohol use. When combined with the liver enzyme test for GGT, the CDT's accuracy rate for detecting alcoholism is 85 to 90 percent.

Steps Toward Treatment

Screening tests are very useful for gaining information about the drinker's behavior, but they are only tools. Concerned family members and loved ones may be tempted to try to interpret the results of such tests, but it's a good idea to leave this to a qualified clinician, whose diagnosis will be an important factor in choosing the right treatment. Such professionals include primary care physicians, psychiatrists, social workers, and addiction counselors. Once a clinician has gathered enough information to make a diagnosis, it's time to take preliminary steps toward getting the person into treatment, such as:

- Medical assessment—Has the person sustained any medical damage from excessive drinking, such as liver problems, injury (from a fight or a traffic accident, for example) or loss of appetite?

Historical Treatments for Alcoholism

Early attempts at curing alcoholism were similar to those of curing mental disorders. Friends and family of a drunkard would put worms and vermin into the alcoholic's drink, hoping that he or she would eventually become disgusted with alcohol. While this method is unsanitary at best, it was one of the first attempts at psychological conditioning.

Another notable attempt at curing alcoholism came in the 1950s, when psychiatrists in Saskatchewan, Canada, came up with the idea of treating alcoholism with the newly-discovered hallucinogenic drug LSD (lysergic acid diethylamide).

- Risk of withdrawal—Based on the frequency and amount of drinking, the physician may want to assess the risk of physical withdrawal symptoms. It would be important to also know how much alcohol is needed for the person to feel its effects, how long since he or she last drank, and if there were previous attempts at quitting that resulted in withdrawal symptoms.
- Medical history—The doctor may want to gather information on any health issues not related to alcohol that could complicate treatment or be affected by drinking, such as impaired blood sugar control for a person with diabetes who is also alcohol-dependent.

In making a referral for treatment, the accuracy of screening tests is crucial so the professional making the diagnosis can match the person with the best treatment. Some doctors might also take an active role in ensuring that the drinker follows through with treatment.

ALCOHOLISM TREATMENT: A HISTORY

From unfounded and bizarre cures to precise treatments, the history of alcoholism treatment has steadily evolved and advanced along with the progress of modern medical sciences in America. However, the recent advent of managed care health systems in the United States has had a profoundly negative effect on the progress of alcoholism treatment, reducing both the physical and monetary resources available and once again calling the utility of alcoholism treatment into question. Sheila Blume, M.D., chairman of the Committee on Treatment Services for Addicted Patients of the American Psychiatric Association, recently commented that "services for people who are substance misusers have been greatly reduced under managed care. As newcomers to insurance coverage, they suffer from being 'last in, first out.' For example, between 1988 and 1998, benefit expenditures for addiction treatment fell by 74.5 percent, while benefit expenditures for general health fell by 11.5 percent." The managed healthcare system has greatly reduced alcoholism treatment and treatment centers, once a booming economic industry in the 1980s.

Modern alcoholism treatments and treatment centers have greatly advanced since the initial diagnosis of alcoholism as a disease by Dr. Benjamin Rush in the 1800s. The initial concerns about alcohol abuse in America were social and had relatively little connection to the detrimental health effects of excessive alcohol consumption. As the eminent French historian and Vice President of the French Government's Commission on Alcohol Jean-Charles Sournia notes in his book, *A History of Alcoholism*:

> Those concerned by the general lack of temperance were few and far between, at best forming small groups . . . drunkenness was upsetting social order in that the lower classes, thought to be the sole indulgers in alcoholic excess, were becoming unruly. It was only some hundred years later that the medical argument became more coherent. Not until the mid-nineteenth century did governments become sufficiently worried to take action; until this time politicians left the subject well alone.

Similarly, Dr. Benjamin Rush used his political connections to raise awareness of the potential health effects of alcohol abuse and began the search for a cure for alcoholism.

Extreme Treatments

The treatments of the time often caused extensive harm and were extremely painful. Dr. Rush would often cut his patients in order to bleed them and cleanse their bodies of the alcohol and similarly would intentionally blister their bodies and purge patients. Even more extreme and dangerous was his use of calomel (mercury chloride) as a laxative. Calomel is a white and odorless toxic solid, which the Environmental Protection Agency says damages the gastrointestinal tract, nervous system, and kidneys and may cause skin rashes and dermatitis, mood swings, memory loss, mental disturbances, and muscle weakness. Such tactics that seem strange to the modern reader were perfectly acceptable in the 1800s and were thought to treat several illnesses in addition to alcoholism. Calomel was a commonly used substance, found in everything from makeup to teething powder.

Dr. Rush also promoted abstinence, a more natural approach to the treatment of alcoholism in the 1800s. In fact, according to Jean-Charles Sournia, Dr. Rush considered cold baths and complete abstinence essential to curing alcoholism. However, this method like others of the time was ill-received largely because it did not consistently produce the desired result, in that people continued to crave and consume alcohol after their treatment. This made it nearly "impossible for Rush to impose his radical therapy in everyday surroundings . . . [and therefore] he proposed the construction of detoxification establishments, asylums and 'sober houses,' where regular offenders would be shut up until cured." These were the first rehabilitation clinics based on a similar logic of those that exist today, namely isolating addicts in a controlled environment where they can receive intensive professional help and focus on overcoming their addiction.

These somewhat peculiar treatments persisted long after the medical career of Dr. Benjamin Rush ended. The early 20th century saw the use of cocaine and morphine as alcohol replacement treatments. The mid-1900s also saw the occasional use of electroconvulsive therapy, which purposefully causes people to experience seizures, as a treatment for alcoholism. Doctors would also intentionally induce hypoglycemia in their patients with the use of insulin, which temporarily impairs the ability of the body and brain to function and can lead to brain damage and even death. None of these treatments truly caught on or became prevalent in the American medical practice, likely because of the great variety of treatment options and the inconsistent results they produced. One "cure" that did develop a national following was known as the Keeley Cure, named after Dr. Leslie Keeley. Dr. Keeley claimed to have discovered a cure for alcoholism, and proceeded to turn this cure into a multimillion dollar company with over 200 treatment centers in the United States that treated more than 400,000 people for alcoholism from 1879 to 1965. The secret to Dr. Keeley's cure was injections of gold chloride, which today is known to be poisonous.

Early Drug Therapies

Several other doctors began to develop drug therapies for the treatment of alcoholism. However, unlike Keeley's Cure these therapies were put forth as treatments and not proclaimed as cures. Moreover, many of the other drug therapies for the treatment of alcoholism in the mid-1900s focused on generating an aversion to alcohol consumption among users. For instance, the drug apomorphine was often given to alcoholics, who, according to Jean-Charles Sournia's book, *A History of Alcoholism*, "were encouraged to drink a quantity of their favorite liquor a few minutes after injection of the drug. The bouts of vomiting induced after this procedure, often repeated on a daily basis, were intended to engender a profound distaste for ethanol." A description of the intended use of apomorphine for the treatment of alcoholism was presented by Norsier and Feldman in the *British Journal of Addiction* and was reproduced by Fredrick Rea in his 1956 book, *Alcoholism Its Psychology and Cure*. The authors describe the treatment as follows:

This technique consists of the injection of apomorphine every two hours, day and night to a patient fasting throughout the treatment, placed in an isolation ward, to whom is administered simultaneously with the injections his favorite alcoholic drink. One begins with doses of 6 mgs and when the patient vomits, this is reduced to 5 mgs until complete aversion and the absolute impossibility of ingesting any alcoholic drink occurs. One then injects every hour during 6 hours, first 4, then 3, then 3 mgs of apomorphine, The following hour we inject 10 units of insulin, and then we offer the patient some sweetened tea and a substantial meal. The duration of the treatment varies from 2 to 10 days according to the case.

Disulfiram or antabuse was used with similar intentions, except that alcoholics were not encouraged to drink after taking the drug. The logic behind the use of disulfiram is classical conditioning, in that alcoholics on the drug will experience many unpleasant symptoms if they consume alcohol while on the drug. The symptoms caused by the interaction of disulfiram and alcohol are not only an altered and unpleasant taste of the alcohol, but also hot flashes, nausea and palpitations. The belief was that this would create a conditioned response among alcoholics not to consume alcohol because of how terrible it made them feel.

Among the mid-1900s drug therapies was the use of magnesium sulphate. Magnesium sulphate began to be used in 1965 with a slightly different logic of how to treat alcoholism. Rather than creating aversion to alcohol through unpleasant physiological effects, magnesium sulphate was used to promote the consumption of water in place of alcohol in the hope that the addict's consumption of water would become habitual and would eventually replace his or her consumption of alcohol. Magnesium sulphate produces a euphoric feeling among humans that is accompanied by great thirst. Doctors would administer magnesium sulphate to alcoholics and then encourage them to drink large amounts of water so the drinkers would "rediscover the thirst-quenching qualities of water."

Lysergic Acid Diethylamide, or LSD, was also used as a potential treatment for alcoholism in the 1960s. It was thought that LSD could help to trigger a change in a person's mental perspective of alcohol consumption. Erika Dyck, professor of the History of Medicine at the University of Alberta, summarized this psychological shift as follows: "The LSD somehow gave these people experiences that psychologically took them outside of themselves and allowed them to see their own unhealthy behavior more objectively, and then determine to change it."

Today, such uses of these drugs, with the exception of disulfiram, are often seen as dangerous and therefore are no longer common practice in the treatment of alcoholism. Furthermore, these techniques have been frequently criticized because they have no direct effect on the desire to drink and only work indirectly through the consequential symptoms produced when the drugs interact with the consumption of alcohol. Nevertheless, these seemingly bizarre drug therapies were relatively common in the mid-1900s and often produced the desired effect of cessation of alcohol consumption.

Drug therapies are commonly used in the treatment of alcoholism, and disulfiram is still currently used as a treatment option. The science between the interaction of disulfiram and alcohol is now better understood, as are the physiological symptoms that result from this interaction. The National Institutes of Health endorse the following description of the symptoms produced by the consumption of both alcohol and disulfiram: The "effects include flushing of the face, headache, nausea, vomiting, chest pain, weakness, blurred vision, mental confusion, sweating, choking, breathing difficulty, and anxiety. These effects begin about 10 minutes after alcohol enters the body and last for one hour or more."

All drugs that are currently approved by the Food and Drug Administration are only prescribed to people who have already quit drinking alcohol. Medications are no longer prescribed to heavy drinkers or used in combination with alcohol consumption as a treatment. There is no medication that is a "cure" for alcoholism, as the only prescribed medications, like disulfiram, are used to prevent people from drinking or to lessen the symptoms of alcohol withdrawal. Naltrexone is another medication that is used to prevent alcohol consumption, but instead of producing adverse physiological effects like disulfiram, it actually prevents the positive feelings often attributed to alcohol consumption from occurring. A third medication that is currently prescribed in the United States for treating alcoholism is acamprosate. Acamprosate functions differently than the other medications in that it actually reduces withdrawal symptoms, such as agitation, headaches, anxiety, nausea, and vomiting, that alcoholics experience when they quit drinking.

Medical Hypnosis

An alternative approach to creating an aversion to alcohol consumption among alcoholics was the use of medical hypnosis. Rather than generating aversion physiologically through the production of undesirable and uncomfortable physical effects, medical hypnosis seeks to create aversion psychologically through practices of unconscious suggestion. Among the largest proponents of medical hypnosis as a cure of alcoholism in the 1900s was the British Society of Medical Hypnotists, which put forth the logic for fighting alcoholism with hypnosis as follows: "Addiction must be fought on its own ground, not on the level of reason and common sense, but in the underworld of the unconscious." The president of the British Society of Medical Hypnotists felt so strongly about this use of hypnosis that he proclaimed that it is an "undisputed fact that hypnosis when properly used can and does cure cases of long-standing alcoholism. It is a fundamental law that what can be caused by suggestion, can be cured by suggestion and, even in all the orthodox treatments, there is a big element of suggestion." The orthodox treatments to which he referred are the commonly used early drug therapies.

In his 1956 review of medical hypnosis aptly titled "Medical Hypnosis" published in the *South African Medical Journal*, medical research JAF Denyssen concludes that

> hypnosis may be regarded as a scientifically established fact. In its application, the directness and economy of effort and time are impressive to both patient and doctor. It offers a rich and promising field for further investigation and research, and should be confined to those subscribing to a recognized ethical code and standard of qualification.

In line with the work of Denyssen, medical hypnosis is still used as a treatment for alcoholism and continues to provide an alternative to drug therapy. For example, an article written in 2005 and published in the *European Journal of Clinic Hypnosis* suggests that the most fruitful use of medical hypnosis in relation to alcoholism is the promotion of the will and desire to quit drinking in people who do not currently possess such a conscious desire. However, medical hypnosis is not commonly accepted in the medical community as an approach for treating alcoholism, and usually isn't part of treatment programs at major rehabilitation centers. Medical hypnosis continues to garner scientific attention in the quest to treat alcoholism.

Inpatient Rehab

Inpatient rehab centers, reminiscent of the asylums of Dr. Benjamin Rush, also remain popular today. For example, what is known as the Minnesota Model of alcoholism treatment began in the late 1940s and is still popular at treatment centers throughout the United States. The Minnesota Model of alcoholism treatment was founded by Dr. Nelson Bradley, a Canadian, working at Wilmar State Hospital in Wilmar, Minnesota. Dr. Bradley's model now entails a complex approach to the treatment of the disease. The Minnesota Model suggests that alcoholism should be attacked from several angles—medical, social, and spiritual. *Courage to Change*, an Aiseiri Research publication on the Minnesota Model, states that recovery from alcoholism requires a change pertaining "not only to the addictive behaviour but to all areas of the individual's life. As such the Minnesota approach seeks to treat the whole person at a physical, psychological, emotional and spiritual level." The Minnesota Model requires a period of residential treatment during which addicts can intensely focus on their own multi-dimensional recovery from alcoholism.

In his 1990 article, "Providing Cost Efficient Detoxification Services to Alcoholic Patients," Nabila Beshai lays out specific processes that are common to all successful alcoholism treatment programs. Beshai states that there are three essential components to the detoxification process that take place at rehabilitation centers. First, the consumption of alcohol must cease. Second, there must be an assessment of the abuser's addiction problems within the context of their life and attitudes. And third, there must be the development and implementation of a rehabilitation program. However, Beshai also acknowledges that this three step process can take place in various settings, such as in hospitals, rehab centers, and homes, and as a result is not limited to residential rehabilitation centers. In fact, according to Dr. Arnold Washton, Director of the Washton Institute on Addictions, there is actually "an increasing demand for outpatient treatment services . . . being created by a combination of clinical and economic factors, including the influx of employed drug abusers who do not need or desire residential care and mounting financial pressure to contain health are costs. To be effective as a primary treatment modality, outpatient programs must be highly structured and intensive and be able to deal with the full spectrum of alcohol and drug addictions."

The original rehabilitation model of Dr. Rush has been greatly diversified to accommodate the individual needs of different people suffering from alcohol addiction. The diversification of alcohol rehabilitation centers has lead to the creation of more than 11,000 addiction treatment programs throughout the United States. With the rising cost of healthcare in America and the decreased federal funding for alcohol treatment centers, nonresidential treatment programs are continuing to grow in popularity.

Treatment for alcoholism has evolved since the days of Dr. Benjamin Rush, when bleeding and purging where common cures for alcoholism. However, more interesting may be the fact that many of the same ideas and principles reoccur throughout the history of alcoholism treatment, namely the use of rehabilitation centers, drug therapy, and relaxation training to treat those addicted to alcohol.

TREATMENT OPTIONS

Alcoholism is complex, and people who seek treatment are unlikely to find a single solution for their drinking problem. Successful treatment usually involves a combination of therapies in order to get and stay sober.

However, alcoholism is more treatable than most chronic diseases, and just about any drinker willing to put the effort into quitting can find the right programs to help.

Although certain recovery groups believe some problem drinkers can make a safe return to moderate social drinking, the goal of most programs is permanent abstinence. The brain chemistry involved in addiction makes moderate drinking a risky gamble for most recovering alcoholics, and there is overwhelming evidence to show that lifelong abstinence is the only sure way to successfully escape the grip of alcohol dependence.

Recent Advances in Treatment

Changes in perceptions about the origins of alcoholism have brought about new thinking in the way the disease is treated. As summarized by the National Institutes of Health (NIH), there have been dramatic advances in the way researchers and healthcare providers treat alcohol dependence and alcohol abuse over the past few decades. For example:

- Thirty years ago, the only medication to treat alcohol was the aversion-therapy drug disulfiram (Antabuse). There are now at least two anti-craving medications available in the United States, with a host of other drugs to treat conditions that are secondary to alcoholism, such as depression.
- In the same time period, only a small percentage of alcoholics received any treatment, and researchers considered alcoholism a disease of middle age.
- Today, researchers can choose from an array of sophisticated screening and intervention tools for early detection and more effective treatment.
- Newer behavioral treatments, such as cognitive behavioral therapy, have given alcohol counselors a better choice of treatment tools.

Researchers have identified genes that can actually put someone at higher risk for becoming an alcoholic, as well as biological markers that make someone less likely to have a drinking problem, such as the "alcohol flush" many Asians experience that makes this population less likely to drink.

Motivational interviewing (MI) is a behavioral therapy developed in the early 1980s. While it has all kinds of healthcare applications related to changing behaviors (such as helping someone with heart disease make beneficial changes to his or her diet), it is particularly useful for treating substance abusers. This is likely due to MI's focus on setting and meeting goals, which can be more practical in the short term than the more exploratory nature of traditional talk therapy.

But with new advances come new challenges, such as dual diagnoses (more than one addiction at a time), medication interactions to watch for, and identifying coexisting emotional or mental conditions that could affect the success of the treatment, all which make it even more complicated for substance abuse care providers to choose the right program. Many factors affect the choice of treatment:

- **Severity of addiction.** People who are alcohol dependent are likely to receive more extensive, immediate, and medication-assisted treatment than those who are identified as alcohol abusers, who may simply need brief intervention and counseling.

- **Coexisting medical or psychiatric conditions**. Some drinkers may enter treatment with health problems related to drinking that may need ongoing secondary treatment, such as hepatitis or other liver problems. Psychiatric conditions could include depression or anxiety, which come with unique treatment requirements, some of which could overlap with alcohol-related treatments, such as counseling.
- **Motivation to change**. The nature of addiction makes most substance abusers reluctant to quit, so it is important to know how motivated the drinker is to accept treatment. Is this the first attempt at getting sober and, if not, what treatment approaches have already been tried? Is there support to help the drinker overcome denial of a problem? Has the person reached some intolerable low point that will make it easier to accept treatment?

The stages of treatment for alcoholism may vary depending on the treatment type, and may overlap between each phase, but in general they follow this order:

- **Intervention**, during which the drinker is screened and diagnosed, and a method of treatment is chosen. The person may need medical attention at this point for withdrawal symptoms or other health problems.
- **Detoxification**, which involves a variety of intensive treatment activities depending on the program, including counseling, behavioral modification, and medications.
- **Rehabilitation**, in which the person works with family, doctors, counselors, and anyone else involved in his or her treatment, to devise a lifelong plan for staying sober.
- **Maintenance**, in which the person must carry out the plan for living alcohol-free. In the same way that a person with diabetes, for example, must vigilantly manage his or her condition, an alcoholic must observe certain lifestyle changes related to his or her vulnerability to addiction. Such changes may include avoiding social settings centered around alcohol, talking regularly with a mentor, and attending support groups.

Brief Intervention

Brief intervention is a form of short-term counseling that is especially useful for alcohol abusers who have not yet reached the dependence stage. It generally involves five or fewer visits with a counselor, who provides the drinker with simple, straightforward information on the consequences of his or her drinking. This is followed by practical strategies and resources to help the person either cut down or quit. Abstinence is always recommended if this approach is used for drinkers who are already dependent.

Brief intervention has been greatly successful in the area of preventing problem drinkers from progressing to alcoholism. It often serves as a wake-up call for many drinkers who didn't previously see themselves as having a problem.

Psychosocial Counseling

Psychosocial counseling helps the brain unlearn harmful thoughts and behaviors that reinforce bad habits, replacing them with more constructive methods for solving problems. Common behavioral treatments for alcoholism include:

Cognitive Behavioral Therapy

Cognitive behavioral therapy (CBT) is one of the oldest and most well-known types of behavioral treatments, with many uses outside of alcoholism treatment, including phobias and anxiety. In an alcohol-treatment setting, the CBT practitioner works with the drinker to identify thinking distortions and negative thought patterns that lessen his or her ability to resist the urge to drink. For example, someone who thinks "the only way I can relax is if I have a drink" needs help in two ways: thinking of other ways to relax and, more importantly, retraining his or her brain to understand that there are other options for relaxing besides using alcohol.

CBT can involve role playing and rehearsal, in which the therapist walks the person through several high-risk scenarios for relapsing, developing practical strategies for getting through these situations without drinking. CBT may also be used to help the person develop coping skills if he or she happens to relapse.

Relaxation Therapy

Anxiety is a common coexisting condition for many people with alcohol dependence. For some, the anxiety was always there, and for others it is a by-product of neurological changes the brain has made to adapt to alcohol's effects. Whatever the reason, anxiety is a powerful force that many alcoholics struggle to overcome without drinking, and the condition can be made worse along with other stressors of quitting, such as health problems or reduced ability to work and support the family.

There are many forms of relaxation therapy to help replace the effects of alcohol. This type of therapy can be especially important for keeping alcoholics from relapsing. Some components of relaxation therapy include:

- Guided visualization
- Meditation

- Yoga
- Aerobic exercise

Relaxation therapy may also provide relief from insomnia, another common problem for people quitting drinking.

Activities Therapy

Often a component of inpatient alcohol treatment, activities therapy can help the drinker restore social and organizational life skills. It works by having the drinker plan and implement activities for a larger group. This provides useful preparation for real-life situations for which the person has lost his or her social skills. It also helps the person visualize how he or she will spend time after rehabilitation treatment, filling the time formerly spent drinking.

Medications for Alcoholism

Currently there is no drug to "cure" alcoholism. The solution for most recovering drinkers is still a long-term commitment to behavioral changes that reduce risk factors for relapsing. However, a better understanding of alcohol's physiological effects on the brain has led to the development of certain medications that can provide vital support for the hard work of recovery.

Disulfiram (Antabuse)

Introduced in the late 1940s, disulfiram is a prescription medication long used as an aversion therapy—that is, it makes drinking so unpleasant that it decreases the urge to drink. It changes how the body metabolizes alcohol by neutralizing a necessary enzyme that breaks it down in the body. Its effects on someone who has consumed alcohol are unpleasant and may include:

- Pain and throbbing in head and neck
- Flushing
- Trouble breathing
- Nausea
- Vomiting
- Profuse sweating
- Racing pulse
- Weakness
- Dizziness

While not a cure, disulfiram is an effective deterrent. It leaves the body slowly, so it works for several days after the drinker ingests it, offering a relatively long period of forced sobriety. However, it can be activated even by nondrinking sources such as cold medications, cooking sauces prepared with alcohol, or chemical fumes containing alcohol.

Anti-Craving Medications

Craving is an area of substance abuse research that provides important clues about what motivates alcoholics to drink—or rather, what prevents them from resisting the urge to drink. As with disulfiram, these medications should not be thought of as a cure but as a supplement to other treatments, helping the person confidently resist cravings until he or she is more able to withstand the pressures of life without alcohol. Anti-craving medications currently available include:

- **Naltrexone (Revia)**. This is a type of drug known as an opioid antagonist, and as the name might imply, it works by blocking the parts of the brain that feel pleasure when a person drinks. In other words, it interferes with the intoxicating effects of alcohol. Although not a complete solution for alcohol dependence, naltrexone is proving to be effective in helping to improve quality of life in many alcoholics. One study published in January 2009 followed the progress of patients taking an injected, extended-release form of naltrexone. Results showed notable improvement in quality of life compared with study participants taking a placebo. Other studies have shown that people who take naltrexone drink less often, drink less when they do drink, and report decreased cravings for alcohol.
- **Acamprosate (Campral)**. Approved for use in the United States in 2004, acamprosate helps alcoholics resist the craving to drink by acting on chemicals in the brain (neurotransmitters). Prolonged alcohol use affects the balance and activity of certain neurotransmitters, such as gamma-aminobutyric acid (GABA). In a recovering drinker, GABA levels are usually low (alcohol increases their effects, so the brain stops making as much), while the levels of another chemical, glutamate, are too high. This imbalance tends to cause excitability and is strongly associated with alcohol craving. Because it dampens this excitability, acamprosate often restores recovering alcoholics' ability to sleep and feel calm. It also poses no threat to the liver, which means it won't aggravate an already overburdened alcoolic liver.
- **Topiramate (Topamax)**. Another potential medication is topiramate, which is chemically related to fructose. Alcoholics who took the drug in studies drank less heavily and could actually abstain from drinking. To date, it is the only medication demonstrated to be effective for alcoholics who are still drinking.

Residential and Inpatient Treatment

For drinkers with the most intensive needs for detoxification (detox) and rehabilitation (rehab), inpatient treatment is often the only option. According to the American Academy of Family Physicians, about 10 to 20 percent of all alcoholics treated for withdrawal symptoms receive inpatient treatment. Inpatient means that the person is temporarily removed from his or her home environment and placed into a facility (such as a hospital or private program) where he or she can be monitored and supported at all hours of the day and night, with no outside influences and minimal contact with friends and family.

As restrictive as this sounds, an immersive environment like this is usually the only way to treat a person who has lost control over his or her alcohol consumption. In many cases, the alcoholic is reluctant to enter this kind of treatment and must be confronted and persuaded by loved ones during an intervention. The drinker may even be compelled by law to enter inpatient rehabilitation if he or she has committed a crime related to alcohol consumption, such as drunk driving or domestic violence. Inpatient treatment is also useful for drinkers whose ability to resist cravings would be overcome by having access to alcohol in the "outside world." Finally, some addicts who are otherwise suitable candidates for outpatient treatment may not be able to travel every day to the facility and would benefit from the residential aspect of treatment.

Types of Inpatient Facilities

While there is no hard and fast rule about the types of inpatient treatment are available, it's useful to consider some broad categories of how to get this kind of help. Types of inpatient treatment include:

- **Residential treatment**—Like it sounds, this kind of inpatient treatment offers temporary residence for people trying to recover from alcoholism or other addictions. Residential rehab centers are generally less clinical and restrictive than their hospital-based counterparts, often providing a serene environment for recovery.
- **Facilities specializing in detoxification**—While many inpatient programs take the alcoholic through the entire process of treatment (from detox to post-rehab support), others focus on this first critical step. Because alcohol withdrawal symptoms can sometimes be medically risky, these facilities offer physician-supervised detox to keep the person safe until he or she can be transferred to a longer-term inpatient treatment program.
- **Hospital settings**—These facilities provide medically supervised treatment for alcoholism and other addictions, offering a combination of medication,

counseling, and other forms of support until the person is ready to live independently and develop a support system for resisting the temptation to drink.

- **Partial hospitalization**—This option is often used to prevent relapse in alcoholics who have completed other forms of treatment. Participants meet several times a week for 4 to 6 hours each time, so it can be considered an intensive form of outpatient therapy. However, it is suitable only for people with a stable home life and a strong support system outside the facility.

- **Adolescent alcohol rehab centers**—Specializing in treatment for teen alcoholics and addicts, these facilities recognize that young people in recovery may find it easier to stay sober by being around others in the same, often bewildering stage of life.

Dispelling Stereotypes about Rehab

The image of inpatient rehabilitation is a common subject of movies and television shows, often depicted as a place where someone goes after hitting rock bottom in a drastic way. While this is how it happens with some drinkers and substance abusers, inpatient facilities are usually different than these portrayals. Most people enter rehab in a less dramatic fashion, and their efforts to stay sober require much more work and long-term commitment than what can be shown in a movie. Some alcoholics find it harder to stay sober and avoid relapse than to stop drinking in the first place, which is why a strong support system and adequate medical care are essential.

In truth, an alcoholic can start recovering from his or her addiction as soon as he or she is admitted into a treatment program. The majority of inpatient programs begin by addressing the person's most pressing needs. For some drinkers, those needs may be as urgent as getting severe withdrawal symptoms under control. For others, it may be medication to restore aspects of their health that have been disrupted by heavy drinking. And some alcoholics have an underlying psychological disorder, such as anxiety or depression, that can complicate the treatment process.

Assessing the Drinker's Needs

To determine someone's needs and how to treat them, physicians and other healthcare providers at inpatient facilities must evaluate each person, physically and mentally. There are many ways to do this, but one of the most commonly accepted methods for inpatient evaluation is to use guidelines outlined in the American Society of Addiction Medicine's *Patient Placement Criteria*.

These instructions were designed to help doctors advocate for the needs of alcoholics and other substance abusers, helping define levels of care. Not only does this help inpatient facilities provide more targeted care, but it allows clinicians to advocate for certain levels of care with insurance companies, who are often resistant to paying for treatment related to alcoholism or addiction in general.

There are separate *Patient Placement Criteria* for adults and adolescents. Each contain five broad levels of care:

- Level 0.5: Early Intervention
- Level I: Outpatient Treatment
- Level II: Intensive Outpatient/Partial Hospitalization
- Level III: Residential/Inpatient Treatment
- Level IV: Medically Managed Intensive Inpatient Treatment

These levels contain an overview of the range of recommended services for the particular level of addiction severity and related problems, such as a disruptive home life, family members or spouses who are actively-using addicts, or coexisting mental illness. Each level of care also contains a description of the recommended type of facility, including the setting, staff and services available, and admission criteria, including if a person is likely to be going through withdrawal symptoms, health problems to look for, emotional complications, receptiveness to treatment (readiness to change), relapse history (if any), potential for a continued problem, and what the environment will be for a person when he or she reaches the post-treatment recovery phase.

During the intake assessment, the inpatient facility's staff will gather important information about the person. This includes behavioral history, such as how much the person drinks, how long he or she has been drinking, and how long since he or she last had a drink. Part of this history may also include coexisting medical or psychological conditions as well as other substance abuse behaviors. A doctor on staff will also conduct a physical exam to find out if the person has other health problems (related to drinking or not), such as liver or pancreatic disease, heart problems like arrhythmias or coronary artery disease, bleeding from the stomach, damage to the nervous system, nutritional deficiencies, or infections. A person may also be asked about his or her family history to determine if there might be addictive behavior that runs in the family. The doctor will also likely take a blood or urine sample to get a complete blood count, liver function test, blood alcohol levels, and electrolyte levels.

One benefit of such exhaustive testing and assessment is to make sure the person's symptoms are attributable to alcohol withdrawal and not underlying physiological issues. Medical conditions that can mimic alcohol withdrawal include abuse of other drugs like cocaine and amphetamines, infections of the central nervous system, brain hemorrhage, poisoning from anticholinergic drugs (often used to treat stomach problems or Parkinson's disease), poorly managed diabetes, or severe hyperthyroidism. A person may even be suffering withdrawal symptoms from other substances that have sedative and hypnotic effects similar to those of alcohol.

Once the initial assessment is completed, the facility staff will determine an appropriate treatment plan. This plan may include medications for such issues as anxiety or withdrawal symptoms, counseling, and all-hours supervision of medically trained staff so that the alcoholic and his or her family can be sure of a secure environment for overcoming the addiction.

About Detox

Once the person is evaluated and a course of treatment decided upon, the first step is usually detoxification (detox). Before a person can begin to receive treatment, he or she first must clear his or her system of alcohol and undergo withdrawal under the controlled supervision of medical staff. There are two main treatment models for detox:

- **Social detox**: In this model of treatment, a person might have only moderate or newer addictive tendencies, making him or her able to go through detox without worrying about major withdrawal symptoms. This type of detox may or may not be medically supervised, and it is most suitable for alcoholics who are very motivated to quit drinking and not heavy drinkers. These people may find success simply by recovering in a supportive environment with others confronting the same issues, with all offering mutual support.
- **Medical detox**: This is likely the most familiar type of detox treatment, as well as the most traditional. Medical detox is often used for long-term heavy drinkers, people in poor health, those with other medical conditions, or people with multiple addictions or dual diagnoses (alcoholism with an underlying psychological condition, for example). It is conducted under a doctor's supervision with round-the-clock care from inpatient facility staff. People who have severe withdrawal symptoms, such as delirium tremens or seizures need medical detox to stay safe and as comfortable as possible during the detox process.

Goals of Detox Treatment

In the detox phase, there are three main treatment goals as identified by the American Society of Addiction Medicine:

- To provide a safe withdrawal from the drug(s) of dependence and enable the patient to become drug-free
- To provide a withdrawal that is humane and thus protects the patient's dignity
- To prepare the patient for ongoing treatment of his or her dependence on alcohol or other drugs

A person may receive medications and other treatment to overcome this challenging step, which can range from uncomfortable to painful to life-threatening, depending on the severity of the addiction. He or she may hallucinate, sweat profusely, feel nauseous, become hyperactive, tremble, or even suffer seizures during the detox phase. A person may also lose the desire to eat, feel irritable, or find it difficult to sleep without the help of medication.

Medications for Alcohol Withdrawal

Alcoholics suffering from the severest withdrawal symptoms may be prescribed a class of medications called benzodiazepines, which have a sedative benefit on the brain similar to alcohol's effect. These medications have been used safely and effectively since the late 1960s and revolutionized the treatment of alcohol withdrawal by directly treating many potential problematic symptoms, such as high blood pressure, increased heart rate, and seizure risk, as well as helping the person stay calm until the worst of the detox symptoms have subsided. Symptoms can start within a couple hours after stopping drinking and last from two to seven days in most cases. Other medications used during detox include haloperidol (Haldol) for hallucinations and beta blockers, such as in people with coronary artery disease whose heart may not be able to take the rigors of withdrawal.

Other Detox Tactics

In addition to medications, inpatient staff members will take measures to keep a person as safe, healthy, and comfortable as possible during alcohol withdrawal. They will keep fluid electrolyte levels stable, sometimes intravenously, because of the fluid loss that often comes from sweating and vomiting. A person might also need nutritional support, especially if the excessive drinking has thrown off his or her habits around normal eating and (nonalcoholic) drinking. This kind of support may include multivitamins and targeted supplements like magnesium sulfate or thiamine. Long-term heavy drinkers are often deficient in thiamine, which can lead to a type of alcohol-related neurological disorder known as Wernicke's encephalopathy.

Post-Detox Treatment

With the urgency of detox taken care of, a person and the inpatient facility staff can focus on the next phase of treatment, which is to address any medical problems brought on by the alcoholic's prolonged heavy drinking. This phase may also include determining how to treat long-term aspects of coexisting psychological conditions that may complicate or even sabotage the alcohol-related treatment. At this stage of treatment, a person's sobriety is fragile and the facility's staff will work to help him or her build a strong foundation for lasting recovery. The hardest work for a person fighting to overcome alcoholism often starts at this time.

The day-to-day work of inpatient treatment is intensive and thorough and it may include individual counseling, periodic psychological assessments and check-ins, support groups, physical recreation and exercise, sober living skills training, and planning for relapse prevention. There may be downtime for reflection and relaxation, and some places may specialize in alternative or holistic activities, such as meditation, guided visualization, and yoga. Other facilities may offer groups specifically for men, women, or teens (although adolescent treatment centers are usually the best option for younger addicts). Certain facilities offer group therapy and other activities that are grounded in a religious or spiritual framework.

During this time, treatment focuses on the whole person and the comprehensive set of factors that led the person to become addicted to alcohol—the same factors that can lead to relapse if not examined thoroughly. In other words, there is more to alcoholism than drinking, as there are conditions that lead up to drinking and those that enable drinking. Therefore, during inpatient treatment an alcoholic may need to undergo additional therapy to address emotional and psychological reasons for drinking. These can include:

- Unresolved childhood trauma
- Escape from the pressures of family and work
- Violent or disruptive relationships, or a household where addictive behaviors are present
- Social or work environments and friendships that revolve around alcohol

Options for exploring these issues include different types of psychotherapy, including cognitive behavioral therapy (CBT), motivational enhancement therapy (MET), and couples therapy, as well as treatment for coexisting addictions and alternative forms of counseling, such as art or music therapy. Group therapy almost always comes into play, and most inpatient treatment programs encourage participation in a 12-step self-help program.

12-Step Programs

One of the most well-known treatment components during inpatient treatment is the 12-step model. Although some 12-step programs are Christian or otherwise religious, many are not faith-based in nature, despite the focus on a higher power. A person undergoing 12-step therapy does not need to self-identify as religious or spiritual to find success through this method—the idea of a higher power is considered a very personal one that does not have to be affiliated with any particular religious denomination. A person's higher power may simply be his or her community of loved ones.

The 12-step model was first proposed by Alcoholics Anonymous in the mid-20th century as the first truly effective method for getting and staying sober. It has since been adopted by many other addicts, including drug users and overeaters, as a mainstay of treatment and recovery. As outlined by the American Psychological Association, the 12-step process involves:

- Admitting that one cannot control one's addiction or compulsion
- Recognizing a greater power that can give strength
- Examining past errors with the help of a sponsor (experienced member)
- Making amends for these errors
- Learning to live a new life with a new code of behavior
- Helping others that suffer from the same addictions or compulsions

By avoiding specific religious or spiritual language, the 12-step method is suitable for people of all backgrounds, ethnicities, and creeds, which may explain its well-documented success. At meetings, the only requirement for attendees is the desire to stop drinking.

Preparing for Life on the Outside

One of the most important goals of inpatient treatment is preparing a person for return to the normal pressures of life, which includes an environment where there is likely to be easy access to alcohol and possibly friendships or social settings that involve drinking. The inpatient treatment staff can help increase a person's chance for successful abstinence by working with him or her to build a foundation of strength and a plan for coping with such temptations.

Options range from medical to therapeutic, and the approach is often multi-pronged. For example, a person may be prescribed naltrexone to cope with alcohol cravings, but this medication is hardly enough on its own. Therefore, he or she may be required to attend Alcoholics Anonymous meetings or some other form of ongoing group support, as well as continued individual counseling. He or she may also return to the inpatient facility as an outpatient to receive ongoing support and therapy.

Finding the Right Inpatient Treatment Program

With literally hundreds of inpatient programs to choose from, it is important to know how to find the right one. For many people, the first nonmedical consideration is figuring out how to pay for treatment. If the affected person has health insurance, he or she (or supportive family members) can usually find an appropriate program on their plan. For uninsured alcoholics seeking treatment, other options may include public health programs or church-based offerings. Payment considerations aside, the following steps may be helpful for anyone seeking treatment:

- Talk with a physician, counselor, or addiction professional and ask for a list of recommended programs. Remember to mention any other additional addictions or psychological conditions, and make sure to find a program that accommodates them, too.
- Contact the inpatient programs that sound promising to see if they are accepting new patients. If they are not, ask them to recommend other facilities. Find out how to enter their program if they are accepting new patients.
- If paying for treatment through health insurance, find out if the treatment facility of choice is covered under this plan.
- Visit the Internet for public health sites on alcoholism, such as the Substance Abuse and Mental Health Services Administration Web site, where provider directories are offered.
- Work with family or other trusted (and sober) loved ones to help find the best program.
- Sign up for the program that makes the most sense. Most insurance companies don't require a doctor's referral in order to enroll for inpatient treatment.

Outpatient Facilities

Some rehabilitation facilities offer clinically managed programs where people can take part in supervised recovery while living at home for part of the time. Some names for these programs include intensive outpatient treatment programs (IOP) and partial hospital programs (PHP). The amount of time a person spends at the facility versus time spent at home depends on the severity of the addiction, how much insurance is willing to cover, the intensity of the program, and the stability of the person. PHPs are sometimes a follow-up step from involuntary psychiatric treatment.

In general, IOPs and PHPs don't handle the detox phase of treatment and require that the person has completed detox before being admitted to the outpatient program. Another requirement is regular attendance at intensive support group meetings.

BARRIERS TO TREATMENT

No matter how bad a person wants to quit drinking, certain obstacles to treatment often exist. Such barriers include:

- The drinker is embarrassed and ashamed to seek treatment because they think they should have enough willpower to quit on their own.
- The person knows there is a problem, but tries to quit on his or her own.
- There is no access to treatment because of low income, lack of insurance, or insufficient insurance to receive only partial treatment, which only gets the alcoholic through the crisis period.
- An incomplete understanding of symptoms, by either the drinker or his or her family and loved ones, which can delay and complicate treatment later on.
- Lack of facilities, such as in rural or developing areas.

Reluctance: When Intervention Is Needed

Many alcoholics are reluctant about entering treatment and may even deny there is a problem. This denial can take place in the face of even the most glaring signs of trouble, such as a job loss or deteriorating relationships. Since every drinker's low point is different, family and friends are often helpless to do anything until the person is willing to seek treatment.

In the absence of being able to force the person to quit drinking, an opposite approach is to conduct an intervention. An intervention should be a collaboration between the concerned loved ones and an experienced addiction professional who can anticipate any problems that could arise. Interventions can be potentially explosive situations when drinkers aren't ready to admit to a problem or feel like the family is "ganging up on" them. However, certain strategies can increase the chances of a successful intervention:

- Make sure the drinker is sober during the intervention.
- Be prepared to document occasions when the person's drinking has caused specific and negative consequences (for example, if the person embarrassed everyone by passing out from excessive drinking in a social situation).
- Cease all efforts to protect the drinker from the consequences of drinking. This includes making excuses, covering up for the behavior, or consistently bailing him or her out from alcohol-related trouble. Most alcoholics will only be motivated to quit drinking if they can experience the full effects of their addiction.

- Make sure the drinker knows that he or she will now have to bear the effects of such behaviors without help, and be prepared to stick with such a plan. This may involve refusing to drive the person to social functions involving alcohol or moving out of the house until he or she agrees to quit.
- Have specific treatment options in place so if the drinker is ready to accept help, he or she can find it right away. This may mean securing a bed in a treatment facility, having a list of counselor's phone numbers ready, or knowing where and when all alcohol abuse support group meetings are within a 10-mile radius of the drinker's home.
- Get as many friends, relatives, coworkers, and loved ones as you can to participate (based on an addiction professional's recommendations). The drinker is more likely to feel supported and accountable with a wider range of concerned people in his or her social circle.

For some alcoholics, the "surprise party" aspect of intervention may feel more like a confrontation than a loving gesture by friends and family members. An alternative to traditional intervention is community reinforcement and family training, or CRAFT (not to be confused with the screening test CRAFFT). This model focuses on supporting the spouse and other loved ones in the alcoholic's community by teaching them how to create a positive environment that promotes and rewards sobriety.

Drinking after Treatment

Some people think part of recovery is not necessarily abstinence, but a return to moderate drinking after treatment. Groups such as Moderation Management and other similar movements argue that not every problem drinker is an alcoholic. While this is an important distinction shared by a number of recovery groups, moderation advocates frequently have looser rules for what defines alcoholism and usually allow members to make their own determination. Since denial is often a central part of alcoholism, most dependent drinkers aren't equipped to make this call themselves. As scientists learn more about the nature of addiction, available information grows to help understand why moderate drinking doesn't usually work for people with alcohol dependence. Over time, even light drinking almost always progresses to addictive drinking, and the drinker must start recovery all over again.

Finding Recovery Online

The advent of the Internet has dramatically changed the landscape for alcoholics reaching out to others for treatment and support. As online resources proliferate more with each year, people who struggle with their drinking behavior can now go online to conduct self-screening, read patient education materials, find a treatment facility, read what others share about certain treatment approaches, and get post-treatment support and resources. While this immediate availability of information carries questionable credibility, the upside is that many alcoholics now feel less alone with their condition.

Getting Help

Someone who drinks too much and cannot or will not quit on their own needs outside help. A trusted friend or loved one, someone who can help assess the person's drinking and assist in deciding what the next steps should be, can be key to a drinker taking that leap toward treatment. Many drinkers use alcohol as a way to cope with pain or shyness, or they may simply be experimenting without considering the consequences. Either way, they are unlikely to seek help on their own.

THE POWER OF ALCOHOLICS ANONYMOUS

For maintaining sobriety long term, no alcoholism recovery group comes to mind as readily as Alcoholics Anonymous (AA). With origins in the Christian temperance movements of the 19th century, AA was founded by a successful young stockbroker named Bill W., whose career had faltered due to his heavy drinking. After being introduced to the philosophy of a religious group called the Oxford Group, Bill W. was able to quit drinking successfully, finding peace, serenity, and lasting sobriety for the first time in his 39 years. In 1935, Bill W. helped another alcoholic, known to AA members as Dr. Bob, understand how sobriety can be achieved through spiritual fellowship with other drinkers, and the two men devoted their lives to helping other alcoholics find the same success.

In the last seven decades, AA has grown from a grassroots network of church groups to a worldwide phenomenon. With countless members and thousands of support groups based all over the world, AA has become the standard of post-treatment support for many recovering alcoholics. The open-door philosophy of AA meetings makes it impossible to know exactly how many people to count as members, but AA uses meeting group reports to estimate that it currently has more than 2 million members.

AA Philosophy

Membership in AA does not require a formal diagnosis of alcoholism. In fact, the only requirement to join is a desire to stop drinking. It doesn't cost money to attend meetings and there are no membership dues, so the organization sustains itself through member contributions. Members may choose to self-identify as being alcohol dependent based on criteria found in AA's guiding literature known as the Big Book.

Rather than making declarations of lifelong abstinence, members choose not to take on a fully-sober future more than one day at a time. For that reason, members do not say they are cured of their alcohol dependence, but instead identify with being "recovered" or "sober" alcoholics who find it much more manageable to live this way.

Another aspect of recovery in AA is the adoption of a sponsor by each new member. The sponsor ideally is someone older, experienced in the ways of AA, and of the same sex.

Sponsors and new members alike find a rich source of ongoing fellowship in AA's self-help groups, which are designed to provide nonjudgmental peer support to help further each drinker's goal of total abstinence. Most meetings occur once or twice per week. Meetings are either open, where members can bring friends and family to hear scheduled speakers or celebrate sobriety milestones, or they are closed, in which only attended by alcoholics.

There are two support groups designed for concerned loved ones of alcoholics. Family members of alcoholics can find support through Al-Anon. Teenagers with parents who are alcoholics are encouraged to join Alateen.

The 12 Steps of AA

The core of AA's recommended path to lasting sobriety is the commonly cited list of 12 steps that offer simple, straightforward direction for drinkers who want to lead sober lives. The steps (see sidebar) are designed to help alcoholics recognize their powerlessness over alcohol and offer a framework for making amends for past alcohol-fueled behavior that may have harmed other people. The steps also focus on building an enduring, meditative relationship with God or one's higher power and maintaining personal accountability.

Faith-Based Treatment

AA's concept of a higher power can discourage people who want to avoid a faith-based system of support during recovery. But AA is not a traditional denominational faith and avoids affiliations with religious organizations. What it does share with many religions is the idea that people (alcoholics, specifically) are helpless on their own, destined to relapse without the support of the community, the 12-step process, and whatever notion of God that makes sense to the individual.

Even so, some drinkers still may reject the thought of relying on a higher power because it may feel like they are surrendering their independence. Or it may feel like a weakness to admit to this kind of helplessness. For those people, AA may not be the best environment, and they may opt for an alternative avenue of treatment. Or, they may choose to rely solely on a more self-directed approach to treatment, such as cognitive behavioral therapy.

The Twelve Steps of Alcoholics Anonymous

1. We admitted we were powerless over alcohol—that our lives had become unmanageable.
2. Came to believe that a Power greater than ourselves could restore us to sanity.
3. Made a decision to turn our will and our lives over to the care of God as we understood him.
4. Made a searching and fearless moral inventory of ourselves.
5. Admitted to God, to ourselves and to another human being the exact nature of our wrongs.
6. Were entirely ready to have God remove all these defects of character.
7. Humbly asked Him to remove our shortcomings.
8. Made a list of all persons we had harmed, and became willing to make amends to them all.
9. Made direct amends to such people wherever possible, except when to do so would injure them or others.
10. Continued to take personal inventory and when we were wrong promptly admitted it.
11. Sought through prayer and meditation to improve our conscious contact with God, as we understood Him, praying only for knowledge of His will for us and the power to carry that out.
12. Having had a spiritual awakening as the result of these steps, we tried to carry this message to alcoholics, and to practice these principles in all our affairs.

The Twelve Steps are reprinted with permission of Alcoholics Anonymous World Services, Inc. (AAWS). Permission to reprint the Twelve Steps does not mean that AAWS has reviewed or approved the contents of this publication, or that AAWS necessarily agrees with the views expressed herein. Alcoholics Anonymous (AA) is a program of recovery from alcoholism only. Use of the Twelve Steps in connection with programs and activities which are patterned after AA, but which address other problems, or in any other non-AA context, does not imply otherwise.

TREATMENT ALTERNATIVES

While the consistent approach and decades-long success of AA may seem like the default treatment for most post-rehab alcoholics, AA is not the perfect fit for everyone. As mentioned, AA's focus on a higher power, while not explicitly touting religion or spirituality, bothers some people who are averse enough to the idea to seek out a more secular approach. For others, talking about their drinking problem, or even attending a meeting with many strangers, is overwhelming and a barrier to successful engagement in AA.

On the other hand, some alcoholics have no problem with AA at all, but they object to other mainstream forms of treatment. Their problem may be with the idea of taking anti-craving or aversion therapy medications to stay sober. Naltrexone, acamprosate, and disulfiram all have extensive, well-documented benefits to report, but each comes with side effects that some drinkers find objectionable enough to seek out alternatives. While not fully accepted by the mainstream alcohol treatment community, some drinkers have found success with alternative methods such as acupuncture, stress management, and hypnosis. In many cases, these treatments are not an "alternative" per se, but rather a supplement to more conventional methods.

Non–Faith-Based Treatment and Support

Treatment options are plentiful for the secular-minded alcoholic and other substance abusers. The following are the more well-known options:

Secular Organizations for Sobriety (SOS)

Uncomfortable leaving their sobriety in the hands of any sort of spiritually designated higher power, alcoholics who subscribe to the ideas of the Secular Organizations for Sobriety, or SOS (sometimes called "Save Our Selves" by its members), choose to rely on a more secular and independent approach to sobriety. Arising from the secular humanism movement, SOS was started in the mid-1980s by founder James Christopher, a sober alcoholic who calls the SOS method "recovery without religion." Similarly, SOS bills itself as an "alternative recovery method for those alcoholics or drug addicts who are uncomfortable with the spiritual content of widely available 12-step programs" and offers the largest non-12-step recovery program available in the world.

Unlike the community-dependent and higher-power-oriented approach of the 12-step method, SOS, like its parent secular humanism movement, puts the power of sobriety into the hands of the individual. Proponents of SOS point out that they do not oppose or seek to compete with other recovery programs, merely that they give addicts an alternative to faith-based programs.

There are some similarities between SOS and AA. Both are nonprofit, with independent chapters and groups all over the United States. Groups are led by nonprofessional leaders, and no membership dues are required (although each group must support itself through member contributions with no outside support). Like AA, SOS attendees need only self-identify as someone seeking recovery and sobriety. SOS also does not take part in matters of politics or other outside matters that may detract from the work at hand, which is to promote sobriety for its members.

Although SOS puts the responsibility for staying alcohol-free on the individual, it emphasizes community support as an essential component for recovery. Group meetings focus on sharing experiences, honesty, confidentiality among members, respect for others, nondelusional thinking, and a rational approach to sobriety, one rooted in the scientific method. SOS also encourages daily affirmations of addiction, a regular acknowledgment designed to derail any denial that may creep into the recovery process (a common culprit in relapse behavior). With this daily admission at hand, the idea is that SOS members are suitably armed in their self-stated, life-long goal of "Sobriety Priority." Although SOS is not a 12-step program like AA, it puts forth a list of similar tenets and goals for its members.

Many secular organizations like SOS have been recognized by hospitals and various court systems as a legitimate and effective alternative to AA and faith-based recovery programs. Thus, people who are ordered to complete a rehab program have an alternative to such religious and spiritual recovery groups. SOS groups are present in every U.S. state and in many other countries.

Self Management and Recovery Training (SMART)

Founded in the early 1990s as yet another secular alternative to Alcoholics Anonymous and other faith-based 12-step programs, Self Management and Recovery Training, or SMART, is based in the ideas of cognitive behavioral therapy (CBT) and the tenets of scientific knowledge and reason. While many alcoholics in a SMART program do hold religious beliefs, and SMART does not bill itself as a replacement for AA as much as a supplement to it, SMART participants focus on an individual, self-motivated approach to staying sober, rather than relying on a higher power. The cornerstone of the SMART method is the program's Four-Point Program:

- Motivation to Abstain—Enhancing and maintaining motivation to abstain from addictive behavior
- Coping with Urges—Learning how to cope with urges and cravings
- Problem Solving—Using rational ways to manage thoughts, feelings and behaviors
- Lifestyle Balance—Balancing short-term and long-term pleasures and satisfactions in life

In fighting urges to drink, SMART participants are given a set of cognitive "tools," such as Vital Absorbing Creative Interest (VACI), Journaling, and Brainstorming, to provide a rational basis for derailing the power of cravings. Since the SMART philosophy views alcoholism and addiction as dysfunctional behavior and not a disease, such tools help participants manage their thoughts and feelings to expose what SMART founders see as "irrational excuses we give ourselves for using," which can easily be reprogrammed into more positive, nonaddictive impulses.

In its short history, SMART has come to be recognized by many mainstream medical bodies as a legitimate and effective means of getting and staying sober. Such groups include the American Academy of Family Physicians, and two agencies of the National Institutes of Health dedicated to addiction: the National Institute on Alcohol Abuse and Alcoholism and the National Institute on Drug Abuse.

Alternative Medicine for Alcoholics

Alternative medicine is a broad category that encompasses several treatment types, including acupuncture, yoga and other movement therapies, hypnosis, herbal remedies, homeopathy, guided visualization, aromatherapy, nutritional support, and even basic exercise. This type of medicine has roots in many cultures outside mainstream medicine, including Native American and Chinese populations. Most forms of alternative medicine are much older than Western medicine, but fail to be taken seriously by some conventional healthcare practitioners, often because the outcomes are harder to measure and are poorly understood by mainstream scientists.

But this form of medicine, as an adjunct or replacement to Western medicine, is growing in popularity with many seeking to improve their health. With lower costs (in most cases), fewer side effects, and a whole-body approach to health (rather than the often reactive, symptom-driven method favored by mainstream medicine), alternative remedies are becoming the subject of government-funded public health studies. A small part of alternative medicine's newfound legitimacy could be attributed to its success in the treatment of people with addictions. Examples of alternative methods for treating alcoholism and other addictions include acupuncture, homeopathy, herbal remedies, and guided imagery.

Acupuncture: Relief from Cravings

The prospect of having one's skin poked with needles fills many people with dread and anxiety, and it may not sound like the most obvious way to resist the persistent pull of alcohol addiction. However, acupuncture is gradually becoming accepted by many addiction professionals as a safe, effective, and even pain-free way to help alcoholics resist cravings and stay sober. Acupuncture is a 2,000-year-old form of traditional Chinese medicine in which practitioners insert tiny needles into various and specific parts of the body to regulate a type of energy known as qi (pronounced "chee"). The idea is that the needles stimulate a process of unblocking vital energy that has become "stuck" due to stress and other ills of modern life and redistributing it throughout the body to restore energy balance.

Proponents of this ancient form of medicine believe that it can be used to treat a variety of health problems, including insomnia, allergies, headaches, premenstrual tension, high blood pressure, joint pain, skin problems, and mood disorders, such as anxiety and depression. Recently, some healthcare practitioners have added addictions and alcohol cravings to that list. A common form of this treatment is called auricular acupuncture, in which needle insertions are limited to the ear. This type of acupuncture may be particularly helpful for general alcohol withdrawal symptoms.

Another kind of acupuncture that has been studied for use in treating addiction is electroacupuncture. Instead of individual needles, this variation involves pairs of tiny needles that are inserted into the skin and then hooked up to a device that sends weak electrical impulses back and forth between the two needles. Electroacupuncture has been tested extensively for use as a pain reliever and as an antinausea and antivomiting agent in chemotherapy patients, and it is also being studied in the field of addictions.

In Chinese medicine's view of alcoholism and other addictions, these kinds of physical dependencies are considered a disruption of the qi. It is believed that acupuncture eliminates cravings by restoring this balance. It is also thought to help clear the brain so that the addict can more ably tackle the issues that led him or her to drink in the first place.

An October 2008 study of electroacupuncture sponsored by the National Center for Complementary and Alternative Medicine explored how this kind of therapy would affect the behavior of alcohol-preferring rats. The rats were given alcohol to drink voluntarily for several days and then were deprived of alcohol shortly thereafter. During the deprivation period, one set of rats received electroacupuncture and another received a fake version of electroacupuncture. Both sets of rats were then given the choice of water or alcohol to drink over the next few days. The rats who received the real version of electroacupuncture were shown to drink less alcohol than the rats who received the fake version of the needling process. While much more research is needed to build on these results, the outcome is encouraging because acupuncture could be considered a good fit for addicts who have tried other means of getting sober. And despite the use of needles, acupuncture is relatively safe and generally free of side effects when performed correctly by a skilled practitioner.

While the effect of acupuncture on alcohol cravings may not be fully understood, it seems easy to understand why it might work (its efficacy is still under review and not fully accepted by mainstream practitioners of Western medicine, such as medical doctors or MDs). If one accepts the premise that acupuncture works, then consider that this therapy treats more than just the physical withdrawal symptoms suffered by most alcoholics—it also relieves related symptoms such as insomnia, depression, and anxiety, all of which can be at the root of problem drinking and can aggravate the detoxification process. By providing a holistic kind of support, acupuncture may treat more than just one discrete part of alcohol withdrawal.

Even the strongest advocates of acupuncture are quick to point out that it should not be the centerpiece of treatment for alcoholism. Rather, acupuncture should be a complementary treatment—never a replacement—for clinically supervised detox and rehab. It should be part of a larger, multifaceted approach that combines all beneficial aspects of Western and alternative medicine, as well as counseling and post-rehab group support, in whatever way that it makes sense for the person trying to get sober.

Herbal Remedies: Natural Detox?

Like acupuncture, herbal medicine has been around for millennia, predating most forms of conventional medicine by centuries. In this type of therapy, prac-titioners, which include naturopaths and herbalists, use plant-based medicines to treat illnesses rather than mainstream over-the-counter drugs regulated by the Food and Drug Administration that many people associate with going to the doctor or pharmacy. Herbs can be used as medications or as supplements to restore a deficiency of some kind. Familiar examples of herbal remedies include echinacea for colds and flu, ginseng to increase energy and stamina, and laven-der as mood-enhancing aromatherapy.

When it comes to treating addiction and alcoholism, herbal medicine tends to focus on cleansing the body of alcohol's toxic effects (therefore giving the liver some relief), as well as supporting the nervous system to relieve the drinker of anxiety and other stresses related to quitting alcohol. Common herbal remedies for alcohol withdrawal include:

- Burdock root, thought to help cleanse the blood during the detox process.
- Milk thistle, used for supporting the liver during the rigors of detox. It con-tains an active ingredient called silymarin, which is thought to keep toxins like alcohol from overwhelming the liver. It may also remove toxins from the liver and help rebuild hepatic cells. Milk thistle is safe and free enough from side effects to be taken by pregnant women.
- Dandelion, often paired with milk thistle because the combination of the two herbs can more potently support the liver than either can alone. Dan-delion may also help stave off alcohol cravings.
- Kudzu, a plant considered a nuisance in some parts of the south, contains properties that dampen the appetite for alcohol, which is a key benefit for drinkers wrestling with their cravings.
- St. John's wort, long used as a treatment for mild-to-moderate depression (especially in Germany, where it has been extensively tested), helps relieve the emotional malaise experienced by many alcoholics, either as a trigger for drinking or as an outcome of quitting.

- Skullcap, catnip, and chamomile, to promote relaxation and calm, which indirectly support the withdrawal process. This may be especially helpful for alcoholics who are coping with nerves and do not want to take a pharmaceutically derived antianxiety medication. Such medications often come with strong side effects that are not present in these herbal remedies.

As with acupuncture, part of the appeal of herbal remedies is their perceived safety and mildness of side effects compared to more conventional pharmaceutical products. However, herbal remedies have chemical properties just like their synthetically derived counterparts, so it is never safe to assume that just because something is plant-based that it can not cause harm. About half of all conventional, FDA-regulated medications are plant-based.

Since most herbal supplements are not evaluated extensively by the FDA yet, using them without a doctor's supervision may mean an ineffective medicine at best and a harmful supplement at worst, especially if it interacts with other medications. For that reason, it is crucial to consult a healthcare provider before taking herbal remedies.

Finally, herbal remedies are supplemental treatments for alcoholism and should never be used without other appropriate components, such as counseling, rehabilitation, anti-craving drugs, and group therapy.

Other Alternative Therapies

Additional forms of alternative medicine are as varied as their conventional counterparts and include:

- **Exercise**—the benefits of regular exercise are well-documented, but most people probably do not think of physical activity as a remedy for getting and staying sober. Exercise relieves feelings of anxiety, a common problem that both provokes drinking and plagues the person trying to quit drinking. It also stimulates the production of endorphins, a much healthier habit-forming substance.
- **Nutritional and vitamin-based therapies**—many people who drink heavily begin to lose their appetite and neglect their nutritional needs over time. By the time they get to treatment, many suffer drastic nutritional deficiencies that can often be corrected with vitamins. For example, thiamine is a commonly given supplement because it is often in short supply in long-time heavy drinkers. This shortage can lead to a type of alcohol-related dementia called Wernicke-Korsakoff syndrome. Other supplements, like amino acids, may help reduce cravings. A low-sugar diet will help restore wildly fluctuating blood sugar levels that come with heavy drinking and detox. To reduce the

population of harmful substances called free radicals, often plentiful in the bodies of alcoholics, some doctors may recommend antioxidant remedies, such as vitamin C, zinc. selenium, magnesium, and beta-carotene.

- **Guided imagery and meditation**—for people who subscribe to the idea of a mind-body connection (that is, the idea that psychological factors can have a significant impact on a person's health), the benefits of guided imagery and meditation are invaluable. For anyone trying to overcome addiction, guided imagery provides a relaxing, yet proactive means for envisioning a life without substance abuse. In both methods, the person sits in stillness, focusing on his or her breaths, while picturing a peaceful place or an aspect of life that will be improved because the person has stopped drinking. They might, for example, picture a healthy, well-functioning liver free from the ravages of alcoholic excess, or a sunny day spent with family without the specter of cravings or unpredictable, alcohol-fueled behavior. Guided imagery and meditation, as with other alternative remedies, effectively promote the relaxation and peace of mind that are vital to a recovering addict.

Alternative remedies, while potentially beneficial, should only be used as part of a larger, clinically supervised detox and rehab program. None of these therapies should be used alone or without proper medical advisement.

4

Alcoholism and Society

The demon of intemperance ever seems to have delighted in sucking the blood of genius and of generosity. What one of us but can call to mind some relative more promising in youth than all his fellows, who has fallen a sacrifice to his rapacity?
—Abraham Lincoln

Alcohol has played a prominent role in the history of American culture and has had a profoundly detrimental effect on millions of American lives. Negative consequences of alcohol abuse stretch far beyond an abuser's body. They touch the lives of the abuser's family and dip deep into Uncle Sam's pocket with decreased economic productivity and rising medical costs.

MORE THAN A DISEASE

Alcoholism is much more than a disease of personal health. It greatly impacts social, familial, and economic situations throughout the United States. It is estimated that more than 100,000 people die of alcohol-related causes each year. The annual cost of lost productivity and health expenses related to alcoholism is more than $100 billion, with millions of Americans abusing alcohol. Alcohol abuse is a disease that kills thousands, ruining families and draining billions of dollars from the economy each and every year.

Whether the cause of alcoholism is genetic, environmental, or social is often contested and debated in medical, academic, and political circles. What is not debated is the reason why discovering the true cause of alcoholism is so important: alcoholism has a tremendously detrimental effect on the economic and social fabric of America. The statistics are grim. In addition to more than 17,000 annual traffic-related fatalities, alcohol abuse in the United States contributes to:

- 1,400 deaths from other alcohol-related accidents
- 500,000 injuries
- 600,000 assaults
- 70,000 sexual assaults

Despite these severe consequences, per capita alcohol consumption in the United States has remained relatively constant over the last 150 years, excluding the Prohibition Era during which consumption was nearly impossible to monitor. In 1850, Americans 15 years of age and older drank 2.1 gallons of alcohol a year. In 2005, the consumption rate was a strikingly similar 2.24 gallons. During this century and a half, per capita alcohol consumption has not changed despite the relatively rapid medical discoveries of alcohol's negative effects and the vastly increasing awareness of alcohol's social consequences.

SOCIALIZED TEENAGE ALCOHOL ABUSE

The trend of alcohol abuse continues to filter down to and dramatically affect American teenagers. There are well over 4 million teenage alcoholics in America— nearly one-third of the total number of alcoholics. A study conducted by Mothers Against Drunk Driving showed that approximately 50 percent of all 10th graders have had too much to drink at some time, and just over 40 percent of 9th graders have reported having tried alcohol at least once. But these experiments come with a price tag—there is a relationship between students who drink and poor grades. In more than 40 percent of students who have academic problems, alcohol is a factor. Alcohol is also involved in 28 percent of all high school dropouts.

Alcohol dramatically affects the social, economic and academic lives of American teens. It can affect the cognitive development of maturing teens, which makes them more prone to alcohol dependence, nervous system damage, and developmental disabilities. Alcohol can damage memory and learning abilities by preventing development of the hippocampus, a complex neural structure in the brain (Youngerman 2005). In addition to cognitive impairments, teens who use alcohol are likely to suffer from vast social and economic consequences. More than 40 percent of individuals who begin drinking before age 15 will develop alcohol abuse or alcohol dependence at some time in their lives.

Where does this cycle start? Teens likely see the behavior of alcohol abuse modeled for them by a parent. Children of alcoholics are at least three times more likely to develop an addiction themselves. And teens today are constantly exposed to alcohol through outpourings of multimedia advertising. Alcohol is everywhere in a teen's life.

Alcohol advertising started in 1996 when the Distilled Spirits Council began advertising on radio and TV for the first time since the 1940s, with many ads targeted toward teens. The Center on Alcohol Marketing and Youth at Georgetown University found that alcohol was advertised on 13 of the 15 shows most popular with teens (Youngerman 2005). Teens tend to enjoy and remember the alcohol commercials more than any other advertisements they see. In a 2002 study, more teens named Budweiser commercials over any other brand's commercials as their favorite (Mintzer 2005). Beer companies spent about $700 million on TV advertising the year of the study. The liquor industry as a whole spends nearly $2 billon a year to say how beer, wine, and booze enhance sex life, reduce cares and woes, and make boring lives more interesting (Mintzer 2005, Ketcham 2000). This may sound like a lot of money, but it pales in comparison to the $166 billion that alcohol-related problems cost the American economy each year. Even worse is the cost in terms of human lives lost to alcohol, as tens of thousands of Americans die from alcohol-related causes every year.

WHO'S DRINKING? ALCOHOLISM IN NUMBERS

According to the 2007 National Survey on Drug Use and Health, more than 50 percent of American adults currently consume alcohol. However, it is important to distinguish between moderate drinking, which can be beneficial for a person's health, and alcohol abuse, which can harm a person's health and others. Sadly, many Americans fall into the latter category as alcohol abusers, as nearly a quarter of American adults binge drink and 17 million Americans are considered to be heavy drinkers. This means that 17 million Americans binge drink more than once a week on average.

Adolescents and Teens

What about teenagers? After all, America has some of the most restrictive laws regulating drinking age in the world, so one would think that the rate of teenage alcohol consumption should be pretty low. However, the consumption rate of American adolescents aged 12 to 17 years has held steady at around 16 percent for the last five years, excluding the entire college age population. This statistic reflects only the drinking patterns of high school- and middle school-aged students, meaning that approximately 1 out of every 5 American high school and middle school students consumes alcohol.

Racial Differences

Breaking the statistics down further by race, white adolescents are more likely to consume alcohol than teens of any other racial group, with a consumption rate of 32 percent. Comparatively, alcohol consumption among African American adolescents was reported at 18 percent in the 2007 National Survey on Drug Use and Health. A significant racial difference is seen in the reported rates of alcohol consumption among American teenagers, with 1 in 3 white adolescents being a drinker compared to only 1 in 5 African American adolescents. The same racial pattern holds true for adult Americans as well, with Caucasian people being more likely to be drinkers than members of any other racial group. Fifty six percent of whites are drinkers compared to 45 percent of Native Americans and 39 percent of African Americans.

By Gender

Among the entire population of American adults, males are more likely to drink than females. Currently, 57 percent of adult American males are considered drinkers, compared to 47 percent of adult American females.

Level of Education

Educational attainment (the highest level of education one has completed) and gender are also associated with specific drinking patterns in the United States. Alcohol consumption rates increase with rising levels of education. The 2007 National Survey on Drug Use and Health found that among adults with less than a high school education, more than 36 percent were current drinkers in 2007, which is significantly lower than the nearly 69 percent of college graduates who were current drinkers. Said another way, people who have completed college as well as people who are in college drink more frequently than people who have not completed college. However, it is important to note that binge drinking does decrease as education increases, which means that college graduates are less likely to binge drink than people who have not graduated from college.

Around the World

How do these rates of alcohol consumption compare to other countries? Do Americans drink more and drink more often than people in other parts of the world? The World Health Organization's Global Status Report on Alcohol in

2004 provided a global context in which to consider alcohol consumption in America.

Comparatively, significantly more residents of European countries drink. The same is true of residents of the Western Pacific, including Australia and Japan. Moreover, Europeans on average drink more than Americans, and Western Pacific residents drink a comparable amount of alcohol. On the other hand, residents of the Middle East are significantly less likely to be drinkers and drink much less than do Americans and Europeans. Specifically, only about 10 percent of Middle Eastern residents from nations like Afghanistan and Pakistan consume alcohol, with the per capita consumption of alcohol in this region at 0.16 gallons. Interestingly, in the Middle East only 1 percent of female residents consume alcohol compared to 17 percent of males. In Western Europe, which includes countries like Britain, France, and Germany, the per capita consumption of alcohol is 3.4 gallons, with 85 percent of the adult-aged population being drinkers. In Western Europe, nearly 16 percent of residents are heavy drinkers compared to less than 7 percent of Americans and approximately 0.1 percent of Middle Easterners. Eastern Europe, including Ukraine and Russia, is often perceived as the region where alcohol consumption is most prominent. Alcohol consumption and abuse rates are in fact slightly higher in Eastern Europe, which has a per capita consumption of almost 4 gallons and a heavy drinking rate of nearly 19 percent.

In the end, Americans do not drink more than their counterparts around the world. In fact, compared to Europeans, fewer Americans drink, and those that do drink consume less alcohol. However, this doesn't mean that alcohol abuse isn't greatly affecting American social and economic life, or that it is causing any fewer problems.

AMERICA'S BAR TAB

The cost of America's seemingly average rate of alcohol abuse is extreme. Current estimates of the financial burden that alcohol abuse imposes on America range from $150 to $300 billion a year. For instance, the National Institute of Alcohol Abuse and Alcoholism recently reported that the U.S. economy loses $185 billion annually due to alcohol-related healthcare and medical expenses, decreased worker productivity, and crime. On the other hand, the Institute for Health Policy reported in 2001 that alcohol abuse by way of traffic accidents, lost productivity, and increased healthcare costs drained $276 billion from the American economy. The lower estimate of $185 billion is more than the federally allotted 2008 individual budgets for the following government departments: Veterans Affairs, Department of Labor, Department of Education, Department of Housing and Urban Development, Department of Homeland Security, Department of State, and the National Aeronautics and Space Administration (NASA). Furthermore, the money that the American economy loses because of alcohol abuse is more than the combined 2008 budgets of NASA, the Department of Education, and the Department of Homeland Security.

The Cost of Alcohol Abuse

The question then becomes, "Who's losing this money?" There is no simple answer. Obviously, individual alcohol abusers are losing money because of increased time off from work, but their particular economic hardships are not included in the national economic effect of alcohol abuse. This statistic, the $185 billion that is included, is solely made up of dollars that the American economy loses or the American government spends as a result of alcohol abuse. The government is forced to spend money on alcohol abuse awareness and prevention, medical costs, legal matters, and law enforcement. For example, more than 50 percent of all homicides and more than 30 percent of all suicides involve alcohol. Conversely, the economy loses money because of lost future taxable earnings due to premature death, lost productivity due to alcohol related illness, and lost productivity due to alcoholism. These consequences of alcohol abuse trickle down to business owners and employers, who are affected in several ways by the negative effects of employees' alcohol abuse. Such abuse affects businesses through higher rates of employee absenteeism, lower productivity, higher health-care costs, and higher employee turnover. In sum, alcohol abuse dramatically drags down the American economy.

Global Effects

Alcohol abuse clearly has terrible consequences not only for individual Americans, but also for America as a nation. Comparatively, a recent report from Ireland states that alcohol related illnesses [in Ireland] have increased by 60 percent in the past ten years. Incidents of alcohol poisoning have increased by 90 percent, and in 2003 alcohol abuse cost the Irish economy nearly $3.5 billion. Scotland reports a significantly higher figure for the cost of alcohol abuse in 2008, listing the net cost of abuse at well over $3 billion. In Europe as a whole, approximately 200,000 deaths annually are attributed to alcohol abuse. More specifically, 25 percent of the deaths of 15-to-24-year-old Europeans males are alcohol related. These statistics illustrate the fact that alcohol abuse is a global problem, yet they are not to be seen as direct comparisons with the United States. Each nation has its own measures and criteria for the cost of alcohol abuse based on their own unique populations and demographics.

Unfortunately, the negative impact of alcohol abuse on the American economy is self-reinforcing. Alcohol abuse drains money from the economy, which contributes to national economic hardship. Then during times of national recession, the level of alcohol abuse in America increases. In short, drinking may contribute to the causes of an economic recession, and in turn an economic recession may contribute to increasing rates of alcohol abuse.

ALCOHOL ABUSE AND THE AMERICAN FAMILY

The effects of alcoholism are in no way limited to the individual alcohol abuser. The dramatic effects of alcohol abuse ripple outward and affect the abuser's family and friends. Often, the most devastating effects of alcoholism fall on children.

Children of Alcoholics

Children of alcoholics are especially vulnerable to emotional, social, and psychological damage by having a parent who abuses alcohol. Children of alcoholics often feel responsible for the pain and suffering that the family experiences and simultaneously develop low self-esteem and mental problems, such as depression and anxiety. Older children of alcoholics may show depressive symptoms, such as obsessive perfectionism, hoarding, keeping to themselves, or being excessively self-conscious. Studies have shown that because children of alcoholics feel they are different from other people, they develop poor self-image, in which they closely resemble their alcoholic parents (Silverstein 1990, Parsons 2003). Furthermore, living with an alcoholic parent can severely inhibit a child's performance at school because of the social instability of his or her home life. Sadly, this unstable home life is often a violent one, with 75 percent of domestic abuse cases involving alcohol. In addition, 30 percent of father-daughter incest cases involve alcohol abuse.

Unfortunately, many American children live in homes with at least one alcoholic parent. A recent survey of Al-Anon members, an organization for the spouses and partners of alcoholics, reported more than 30 percent of their members have at least one child living at home. This means that at least one in three alcoholics have children. The ways of alcoholic parents often rob a healthy childhood experience and normal development from their children, replacing it with social uncertainty and mental instability. Children of alcoholics are often caught in a battle between their parents and alcohol, all too often lost in the middle and disengaged from their family. Children often have just as much difficulty relating to their nonalcoholic parent as they do to their alcoholic parent. Alcoholism tears American families apart, often creating a massive crack through which American youth fall.

When Children of Alcoholics Grow Up

The dramatic effect of having a parent who abuses alcohol does not end after a child comes of age, but often persists into that child's adult life. The effect of having an alcoholic parent manifests itself within the now adult-aged child in the form of depression, aggression, and an inability to develop stable relationships. Adult-aged children of alcoholics may also have difficultly maintaining a quality family environment for their own children because their alcoholic parent was irresponsible and didn't provide them with basic children's needs (Parsons). In this way, the familial effect of alcohol abuse appears to be not only persistent but cyclical, in that the children of alcoholics develop similar mental and social problems regardless of their own level of alcohol use.

Alcoholism does not only affect the alcohol abuser, but it may also affect several generations of the abuser's family. Even worse, it appears that within a family environment, alcoholism is a self-reinforcing family disease. Family members adapt and become accustomed to living with an alcoholic. In this way, the alcoholic home becomes normalized and more functional options are not contemplated.

Al-Anon and Alateen

How can this detrimental cycle of alcoholism's effects on the family be stopped? Just as there are organizations set up to help alcoholics recover, there are organizations for the parallel recovery of the family members of alcoholics. Alcoholics Anonymous (AA) has given rise to two such organizations: Al-Anon and Alateen. Both of these organizations are based on the structure of AA, with the first designed to aid spouses of alcoholics and the latter aimed toward helping children of alcoholics. The general idea behind Al-Anon and Alateen is to help members return to a normal family life. This is accomplished through members sharing experiences that provide alternatives to the alcohol-dependent home. Al-Anon and Alateen are centered around anonymous group meetings at which members share their stories and cultivate each other's recovery. The organizations state that:

> Members share their own experience, strength, and hope with each other. You will meet others who share your feelings and frustrations, if not your exact situation. We come together to learn a better way of life, to find happiness whether the alcoholic is still drinking or not.

It is this exposure to a different way of life that Al-Anon and Alateen hope will help spouses and children of alcoholics to break the pattern of progression that alcoholism has on their families. A 2006 survey of members indicated that more than 80 percent of members believe their mental health and well-being was much improved due to Al-Anon. A similar survey of Alateen members indicates that most members' health, well-being, and daily functioning greatly improved due to Alateen.

DRUNK DRIVING

Far too many Americans think they can drive safely after drinking, only to end up hurting themselves and thousands of other people each year. Recent surveys estimate that approximately 13 percent of Americans have driven while intoxicated in the last year. This equates to millions of individual drunk drivers on the road over the last year, without accounting for repeat offenders. Among 18 to 25 year olds in 2007, the rate was significantly higher. Nearly 23 percent of Americans in this age group reported that they have driven under the influence of alcohol within the past year. Residents of Wisconsin were most likely to report driving under the influence, with over 26 percent of the state's population confessing to driving drunk, while Utah residents were the least likely to drive drunk, with just under 10 percent of the population admitting to driving while intoxicated. Driving under the influence of alcohol is clearly an age-related phenomenon, with the highest percent of drunk drivers being from 21 to 25 years of age. The percentage of Americans driving drunk increases until the age of 25, after which the percent tapers off.

Traffic Deaths Due to Alcohol

The millions of instances of drunk driving in America lead to more than 17,000 alcohol-related traffic deaths each year. This translates to approximately 36 people being killed and 700 injured daily in alcohol-related traffic accidents. These preventable deaths account for more than one-third of all traffic fatalities in America. There are thousands of nonfatal alcohol-related traffic accidents each year as well. The total price tag of alcohol-related traffic accidents for American tax payers is over $50 billion annually. The job of stopping drunk driving and lowering the human and economic costs of driving drunk lies largely with individual Americans who have the choice and responsibility to not drink and drive.

Under-the-Influence Arrests

Unfortunately, law enforcement agencies in America are ill-equipped to stop every drunk driver. The Centers for Disease Control and Prevention reports that in 2007 more than 1.4 million drivers were arrested for driving under the influence of alcohol or narcotics, which is less than 1 percent of the 159 million self-reported episodes of alcohol-impaired driving among U.S. adults each year. This means that law enforcement officers are largely outnumbered by drunk drivers, and that individual Americans must take control of drunk driving.

Considering the inability of law enforcement officers to stop every drunk driver, police departments are developing innovative tactics to expand their presence, and states are enforcing stricter penalties in hopes of reducing the number of drunk drivers on the road. Police are starting to implement sobriety checkpoints, which are instances when law enforcement officers will randomly stop drivers to check their blood alcohol content in hopes of raising awareness and deterring motorists from drinking and driving.

The Penalties for Driving Drunk

The possible penalties for drunk driving now include jail time, probation, an automobile ignition lock that tests the blood alcohol content of the driver, special license plates that indicate a driver has been convicted of driving under the influence of alcohol, and community service. However, these are only the legal penalties. Drunk drivers also often face penalization from employers and auto insurance companies. Depending upon their occupation, convicted drunk drivers are often fired. They can also lose their automobile insurance and in turn their right to drive.

The fines and jail sentences associated with drunk driving convictions can more than double for an individual's second offense. However, the legal fallout from a drunk driving conviction varies widely by state, and there are only two national stipulations against drunk driving: the zero tolerance law and the national blood alcohol content of .08. The zero tolerance law stipulates that it is illegal in all states for anyone under the age of 21 to operate a motor vehicle with a blood alcohol content above .00.

Drunk Driving and the Law

Drunk driving legislation has an interesting history in America, with the first law against driving while under the influence being established in Indiana in 1939. This law made it illegal for an individual to operate a motor vehicle with a blood alcohol content of .15 or more, which is nearly double the current national limit of .08. In many states, the first legal limit was .20 or .15, with 39 states having laws pertaining to drunk driving by 1963.

Interestingly, the Road Safety Act of 1967 in Britain established a national blood alcohol content limit for driving at .08. Similar laws limiting the blood alcohol content of legal drivers to .08 were established in Australia in 1961, in Canada in 1969, and in Germany in 1973, where the legal blood alcohol content for drivers has since been lowered to .05. The current .05 blood alcohol limit of Germany is surpassed only by Sweden, which has a legal blood alcohol limit for drivers at .02, which is one-fourth of what is considered legally acceptable in the United States. It was not until the 1980s—nearly two decades after Britain passed the Road Safety Act—that the United States began to lower its legal blood alcohol limits to .10. The national legal alcohol limit in the United States was established by Congress in 2000 due to heavy pressure from Mothers Against Drunk Driving.

This makes for an interesting international comparison in that Europeans and Americans have relatively similar drinking habits, yet European nations have significantly stricter laws regulating driving under the influence of alcohol. Adding to this comparison is the effects that lowering blood alcohol limits has had in America, with decreasing trends in the number of fatal accidents for teenagers over the last 20 years. Increased awareness of the problem of drunk driving, stricter legislation regulating driving under the influence, and more aggressive law enforcement have all helped with this trend. More specifically, it has been found that lowering the blood alcohol limit from .10 to .08 corresponded to approximately a 7 percent decrease in alcohol-related traffic fatalities, which means that nearly 500 lives are saved every year. These findings have sparked talk among activists of lowering the legal limit to .05.

DRINKING AND YOUNG PEOPLE

There is no country, socioeconomic class, or age group that has not been affected by alcoholism and alcohol abuse. While most people who drink do not have a problem, the relatively small percentage of those who will develop an alcohol use disorder adds up to millions. For example, according to the American Academy of Family Physicians, 3 out of 4 adult drinkers suffer no ill consequences, and even though much of the remaining 25 percent manage to get their drinking under control before becoming addicted, a large number of them will develop a dependence on alcohol. By some estimates, about 8 to 10 percent of the population will develop an alcohol use disorder, and the figure is higher for those under age 25.

For the relatively small percentage of addicted drinkers, the effects can be devastating. This is especially true for young people in adolescence through the college years. With no frame of reference for understanding the effects of drinking, young people are more vulnerable to the consequences of alcohol abuse.

According to the Centers for Disease Control and Prevention, young people who drink—especially binge drinkers—are more likely to experience these problems:

- School problems, such as higher absence and poor or failing grades
- Social problems, such as fighting and lack of participation in youth activities
- Legal problems, such as arrests for driving or physically hurting someone while drunk

- Physical problems, such as hangovers or illnesses
- Unwanted, unplanned, and unprotected sexual activity
- Disruption of normal growth and sexual development
- Physical and sexual assault
- Higher risk for suicide and homicide
- Alcohol-related car crashes and other unintentional injuries, such as burns, falls, and drowning
- Memory problems
- Abuse of other drugs
- Changes in brain development that may have lifelong effects
- Death from alcohol poisoning

Alcohol and Behavior

What is it about drinking that leads to such problems? Alcohol affects the brain and leads to these complications:

- Impaired judgment, which can cause people to behave more recklessly than they would if they weren't drinking
- Lowered inhibitions, leading to behaviors that the drinker may regret later (like having sex with someone they don't like or revealing things about themselves that they otherwise wouldn't)
- Impaired memory, which can cause a form of alcohol-related amnesia known as a blackout, as well as longer-term memory loss

The developing teenage brain is even more vulnerable to these impairments, making young drinkers more likely to make poor decisions and suffer long-term effects (see Figure 4.1). And the problem extends beyond the teen years—new research shows that the human brain continues to develop until age 25 and that the developing brain is more vulnerable to the effects of alcohol than the mature brain. A person who doesn't drink until age 21 is five times less likely to develop alcoholism than someone who starts drinking at or before age 14 or earlier.

Making Smart Choices

High school and college students commonly find themselves in social situations involving alcohol, often making the decision to drink or not without adult supervision. According to the Substance Abuse and Mental Health Service Administration, kids who talk with a parent about the dangers of drinking have lower rates of alcohol use than those who don't. These kids are more likely to make smart choices when around alcohol and resist peer pressure to drink.

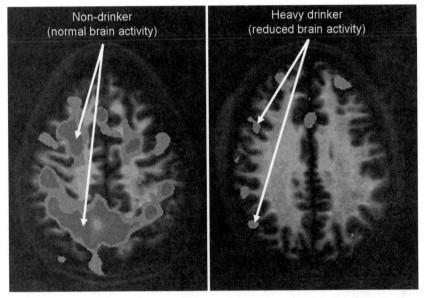

Figure 4.1 The brain of a 15-year-old heavy drinker (right) is significantly less active than the brain of a 15-year-old non-drinker (left). [Courtesy of Susan F. Tapert, PhD, University of California]

ON CAMPUS: UNDERAGE AND UNDER THE INFLUENCE

Similar to drunk driving in the 1980s and 1990s, binge drinking on college campuses has recently garnered much public attention raising awareness of the prevalence of underaged drinking at American colleges. The demographic breakdown of college drinkers is a microscopic version of the demographic picture of America as a whole, namely with white males as the most frequent drinkers. Accordingly, black colleges and all women's schools historically have lower rates of alcohol abuse, while drinking is more common at colleges with fraternity and sorority systems and at colleges with an emphasis on varsity athletics.

How extensive is drinking on college campuses? According to the 2007 National Survey on Drug Use and Health, nearly two-thirds of American college students drink and slightly less than half binge drink. Even more troubling is the fact that young adults aged 18 to 22 enrolled full time in college were more likely than their peers not enrolled full time to have used alcohol in the past month, binge drink, and drink heavily. Considering the entire population of college students in America, 2 out of 5 will be binge drinkers, two more will be moderate drinkers, and only one will abstain from alcohol consumption.

This means that young adults who attend college are more likely to abuse alcohol than their working peers. Research indicates that not only are college students more likely to binge drink than their working peers, but that college students were less likely than their working peers to be drinkers before attending college. Something takes place in the college environment that turns many nondrinking teenagers into drinkers and some nondrinking teenagers into alcohol abusers.

Several factors are likely interacting to cause this increase in both drinking and binge drinking at college. First, the peak age for alcohol consumption in America is in the early twenties regardless of an individual's educational background. Second, at college there may be a critical mass of peers that convince certain young adults to drink or binge drink who may have otherwise abstained from alcohol and avoided alcohol abuse. Third, in the college environment there is frequent social interaction between students legally old enough to drink and those who are not, which may encourage underage students to drink. Lastly, research has documented that college students often have a distorted perception of how much alcohol is actually used and abused on campus, which leads them to believe that it is normal to drink, and even acceptable to binge drink. Drinking becomes perceived as part of the college culture and a student's common college experience.

This normalized drinking behavior is having a dramatic impact on America's college youth, with alcohol being reported as a primary cause of academic problems by approximately one fourth of all college students. Approximately 1,700 college students die every year from alcohol-related accidents, and thousands more are injured. Alcohol is a leading cause of violence among college students, especially sexual assaults. College-aged students who use alcohol are also significantly more likely to use other illegal drugs than their nondrinking peers. The probability of a person using illicit drugs increases as the level of that person's drinking increases, and the same pattern holds true for alcohol and tobacco use.

The detrimental effects of alcohol abuse are present throughout American society, affecting each and every demographic category of the American population—educated and uneducated, young and old, black and white. The widespread reach of alcoholism touches nearly every aspect of American society, from college culture to the American economy, and from the stability of the American family to the health of individual Americans.

5

Alcoholism-Related Problems

The problem of alcoholism has broader, more indirect effects that are not limited to the personal health and life of the drinker. It is obvious a woman can't get pregnant from drinking a beer, for example, but the alcohol in the beer can lower her or a certain male's inhibitions enough for him or her to have unprotected sex, which can lead to unwanted pregnancy. A cocktail alone usually is not the subject of disagreements, but drinking too many of them can impair judgment and make a person more aggressive and prone to picking fights, which leads to a more violent world. The trickle-down problems of alcohol abuse are numerous, widespread, and devastating to millions of lives.

ALCOHOL, VIOLENCE AND CRIME

For as far back as historians can trace, abusing alcohol has gone hand in hand with abusing authority and abusing others. Alcohol abusers often tend to hurt themselves, hurt the ones they love, and hurt the law enforcement and judicial systems for everyone else.

Violence

The combination of impaired judgment and lowered inhibitions is a potent one for aggressive people who drink. These effects play a huge role in the tendency to start fights, commit acts of sexual assault or domestic violence, or intimidate others. The association between alcohol and violence is supported by compelling statistics from the National Institute on Alcohol Abuse and Alcoholism (NIAAA). Violent offenders who drank at the time of their offense made up:

- 86 percent of homicide offenders
- 37 percent of assault offenders
- 60 percent of sexual offenders
- 57 percent of men and 27 percent of women involved in marital violence
- 13 percent of child abusers

Drinking also makes a person more vulnerable to being a victim of crime. Why the association between alcohol and violence? There is no universally accepted explanation, but many theories exist, including the idea that alcohol's tendency to impair judgment makes aggressive people less likely to understand the risks of committing acts of violence, which include injury, hurting a loved one, and spending time in jail. Alcohol's dampening effect on the brain chemical serotonin, which is believed to have an inhibiting influence on behavior, may also lead to the increased aggression and impulsiveness that makes some drinkers violent.

There may also be more indirect associations between alcohol and violence. For example, young men who engage in antisocial behaviors like fighting and hostility usually have higher levels of testosterone, a hormone that accounts for traits like competitiveness and aggression. One NIAAA study found that alcohol consumption increased aggressive behavior in squirrel monkeys with high levels of testosterone and not in those with low testosterone.

Alcohol and aggression may simply stem from similar impulses in some people. In other words, someone who is prone to risk-taking behavior may express that trait in all sorts of ways, which may include heavy drinking, thrill-seeking activities like fast driving, and fighting. Similarly, children from violent or abusive homes are at a higher-than-normal risk for many risky behaviors, including heavy drinking and fighting.

Conversely, people who drink are also more likely to become victims of violence. A 2006 study published in the *Journal of Adolescence* reported that young adults who consume alcohol were more likely to be hit than their adolescent counterparts who did the hitting.

Crime and Criminal Behavior

In addition to many drinkers' tendency to be violent, alcohol can lead to other destructive behavior, namely criminal activities. The most common of these is driving under the influence of alcohol or other drugs, which caused 13,470 deaths in 2006, according to the Centers for Disease Control and Pre-

---

Preventing Alcohol-Related Violence

If you choose to drink, there are things you can do to help avoid violence:

- Don't drink on an empty stomach — alcohol has stronger effects on someone who hasn't eaten first.
- Know your limits and how drinking affects you — it may make you feel and do things out of the ordinary, like such as start fights or become less likely or to be able to protect yourself in a violent situation. Resist peer pressure to drink more than you're comfortable with.
- Don't drink more than one alcoholic beverage per hour.
- If you're in a social situation where people are becoming aggressive, don't stick around.
- Avoid being alone or secluded with anyone you don't know, especially if sex is involved.
- Don't use alcohol to cope with pain or anger — get help in other ways, such as talking with friends or family.
- Avoid socializing with anyone who carries a weapon or engages in violent behavior, such as someone in a gang.

---

vention. This accounted for a third of all traffic fatalities that year. Other alcohol-associated crimes include assault, rape, child abuse, theft, and illicit drug use.

Alcohol use among young people is often an early predictor of criminal behavior later in life, an idea supported by studies such as the 2003 report in the journal *Pediatrics* that revealed that underage drinkers often go on to use illicit drugs, commit theft, and drive drunk. Among criminal offenders participating in a 1998 Bureau of Justice survey, 40 percent reported that they had been drinking at the time of their offense.

As with other problems related to alcohol use, drinking's effect on the brain is a primary factor for bad behavior. The high that many people feel after one or two drinks can be replaced by more troublesome effects after prolonged alcohol consumption, including mood changes, poor impulse control, slowed reaction times, and impaired judgment. These changes in brain chemistry are what make some people think they can handle drinking and driving, get away with shoplifting, or start fights without negative consequences.

Family Problems

Spouses, partners, children, and friends are usually the most commonly affected people in the life of an excessive drinker, and they are often the people pushing the alcoholic into treatment (the nature of addiction makes it nearly impossible for the drinker to seek help voluntarily). Not everyone who drinks excessively is an addict, but any form of alcohol abuse can wreak havoc on family and social relationships. Effects on these relationships can include:

- Emotional distance, such as if the drinker is using alcohol to cope with personal problems and doesn't want to tell anyone.
- Violent behavior, including physical or sexual abuse.
- Sexual problems, such as when excessive drinking interferes with the physical and emotional aspects of intimacy.
- Legal problems that can affect the whole family.
- Obnoxious or aggressive behavior when the drinker is intoxicated, which can disrupt get-togethers or cause public embarrassment.
- Financial problems, such as if the drinker is missing days at work because of hangovers, or if a family needs to pay for alcohol treatment.
- General disharmony among family members or friends whose ability to connect emotionally with the drinker is compromised.

Family and other loved ones can be the most important factor in helping a problem drinker get help because these people are often heavily influenced by such relationships. However, friends and relatives can also contribute to the problem if they abuse alcohol themselves, encourage heavy social drinking, or ignore the problem as well.

Domestic Abuse

Domestic abuse involves many types of offenses, including hitting, slapping, forced sex, pushing, verbal or mental abuse, forced isolation, or any kind of coercion, such as threatening to harm the children. The relationship between domestic abuse and substance abuse is a complicated one. While it's not necessarily true to say that drinking causes domestic abuse, the association between them is undeniable.

For example, in 1999 the *New England Journal of Medicine* concluded that women at the greatest risk for injury from domestic violence included those with male partners who drank excessively or used drugs—those women were 3.6 times more likely to be assaulted by their partners. In a survey of domestic violence victims, the U.S. Department of Justice reported that 75 percent of incidents involved an offender who had been drinking. Clearly there is a link between drinking and domestic abuse, but is it accurate to identify alcohol as the cause?

Because many batterers learn the behavior at an early age, drinking is seen by many domestic violence experts be more of an intensifying factor than an actual cause. It may be more accurate to view drinking and partner abuse as overlapping problems, because they need to be treated separately in order for the offender to stop the abusive behavior. In other words, a batterer who is treated for a substance abuse disorder is unlikely to stop hitting if he or she isn't also in a program to curb the violent behavior. Furthermore, many abusers use alcohol as an excuse for their behavior, which incorrectly relieves them of the responsibility for their actions and could give them a reason not to seek treatment for their offenses.

Suicide

Another form of violence is suicide, and anyone who drinks excessively may be at a higher-than-normal risk. In a 2002, Substance Abuse and Mental Health Services Administration found that 28 percent of suicides among children aged 9 to 15 were attributable to drinking. Reasons why include:

- Alcohol can exacerbate mood disorders like depression, making a bad situation even riskier.
- Alcohol skews a person's judgment, making him or her less likely to think clearly and envision a hopeful future. In fact, drinking may reinforce the thinking distortions that plague suicidal young people, such as "Nobody understands me" or "I'll never feel better."
- Someone who drinks excessively, especially if using alcohol to cope with emotional problems, may also neglect other aspects of their health, such as proper nutrition and adequate sleep, which make them more vulnerable to the effects of depression.

According to some researchers, the link between drinking and suicide is similar to that of alcohol and violence. Alcohol's inhibitory effect on serotonin and other brain chemicals (neurotransmitters) leads to poor impulse control, which means someone contemplating suicide is more likely to try it if he or she has been drinking.

ALCOHOL AND RISKY BEHAVIOR

One of the most common effects of drinking is lowered inhibitions and impaired judgment. These are common factors in risk-taking, especially among young drinkers, who are at a phase of life where they are exploring many new experiences and often trying alcohol for the first time. According to a survey of almost 4,000 students in 8th to 10th grade published in *Alcohol Health & Research World*, alcohol was more likely to be associated with these risky behaviors:

- Fighting or carrying weapons
- Having unprotected sex or having sex with strangers

- Going to places that are known to be dangerous
- Talking to strangers
- Letting people see how much money the respondent was carrying
- Going on a blind date with someone the respondent hardly knew
- Hitchhiking
- Walking alone through unsafe neighborhoods, or walking outside alone late at night
- Riding on empty buses or train cars
- Driving recklessly, driving under the influence of alcohol, or riding in a car where the driver has been drinking

Binge Drinking

One of the most dangerous of risky behaviors involves alcohol consumption itself. The practice of binge drinking is unfortunately common among adolescents and college students. Many people have witnessed firsthand one or more instances of binge drinking, such as at a party where someone consumes several drinks in a very short time. The official definition of binge drinking is having five or more drinks (four or more for women) in a row within a two-hour period.

Binge drinking is especially common in the military and on college campuses, where many young people celebrate their newfound independence before their judgment is developed enough to make smart choices. Being away from home for the first time, they may engage in heavy bouts of alcohol consumption without having the experience or common sense to know they're putting themselves in danger. Binge drinking is clearly not a smart choice—overloading the body with too much alcohol can lead to further risky behaviors such as unprotected sex, fighting, and drunk driving, as well as numerous health problems. At its worst, it can lead to accidental and catastrophic injuries, such as from a fall, and alcohol poisoning, which can cause seizures, vomiting, and death. Signs of alcohol poisoning include disorientation, pale or bluish skin, slow or labored breathing, and unconsciousness.

Sexual Problems

Under normal circumstances, neither drinking nor sex is unhealthy or unsafe between consenting and responsible adults. But people under the influence of alcohol can make foolish choices about sexual behavior, which can lead to serious, lifelong consequences. These outcomes can include unwanted pregnancy, sexually transmitted diseases (STDs), and a damaged reputation. Perhaps the

21st-Birthday Binge Drinking

A prevalent custom among college students is to drink heavily on the day they turn 21. In a survey conducted by the University of Missouri, 83 percent of students drank on their 21st birthday, with 24 percent of women and 34 percent of men consuming more than 21 alcoholic drinks. With immediate concerns about passing out, hangovers, and alcohol poisoning aside, a 21st birthday binge promotes heavy drinking at other celebrations, increasing the risk for alcoholism.

most devastating outcome is sexual assault, which is often associated with alcohol use by both victims and perpetrators.

Effects on Sexual Performance

Alcohol's effects on sexual performance are multifaceted. Because of alcohol's relaxing effects, people who drink are more likely to be sexually active. Conversely, it can also cause impotence and decreased sexual pleasure by interfering with circulation and nerve impulses.

Many people think alcohol is an aphrodisiac (a substance that increases sexual drive), even though there is no hard evidence to support this theory. The root of the idea probably has more to do with alcohol's ability to inhibit the brain's excitatory centers (in other words, in small amounts it helps some people relax). But people who drink excessively before having sex are less likely to perform well, stay awake, or fully remember the experience later on.

Sexual Assault

Lowered inhibitions and impaired judgment can be a dangerous combination when men and women drink excessively together. Scenarios of how unchecked alcohol consumption can lead to sexual coercion include:

- A man and woman engage in kissing or other sexual behavior, and the woman changes her mind. The man, whose aggression may be fueled by alcohol, doesn't want to stop and forces the woman to have sex. This is sometimes known as date rape.
- A man feels rejected, bitter, or sexually jealous, and his feelings are intensified by the effects of alcohol, which makes him more aggressive. He acts on his aggression by forcing a woman (perhaps his own partner) to have sex with him.
- Some men in social settings involving alcohol imagine that women who drink are more likely to want sex, so they coerce them into it.

- Men in emotionally volatile relationships may imagine their partner is cheating or otherwise humiliating them and act on their sexual jealousy by committing an act of alcohol-fueled assault.
- A man slips a date rape drug into a woman's drink at a party. Because the effects of such drugs can resemble those of drinking, the woman may appear to be drunk and only the perpetrator knows she's been drugged. Once the woman is under the influence of this kind of substance, the man takes advantage of her by having nonconsensual sex that she may not remember the next day.

Female college students are especially vulnerable to drinking-related sexual assault, particularly in schools where socializing takes place at parties and bars. The number of such alcohol-fueled attacks is hard to estimate. Women often don't report them because they are scared of their assailant or ashamed because the encounter started out consensually. Some women may not even be aware that they've been raped or otherwise sexually coerced because they don't know the legal definition of sexual assault, which includes any sexual behavior a person doesn't agree to, such as vaginal or anal intercourse, forced oral sex, and attempted rape. Some women may blame themselves for an imagined role in the attack, such as drinking too much or trusting someone they didn't know very well.

Despite the lack of precise facts and figures, the prevalence of alcohol-related sexual assaults on campuses is higher than most people would guess. For example, the National Institute of Alcohol Abuse and Alcoholism estimates that half of all female college students have been sexually assaulted and that half of those attacks involved alcohol consumption. The American Medical Association estimates that drinking by college students contributes to 70,000 sexual assaults or date rapes each year.

Unprotected Sex

However, most sexual encounters involving alcohol are not sexual assault. Many couples use alcohol as a way to relax and enjoy social settings or physical intimacy. Even casual sex is consensual most of the time. However, even among willing sexual partners, the influence of alcohol can cause lapses in judgment or a sense of urgency that prevents them from using some form of protection to prevent pregnancy or sexually transmitted diseases. A 2002 study by the Kaiser Family Foundation yielded these statistics about young people aged 15 to 24, alcohol, and sexual behavior:

- About a third of young people who participated in the study stated that alcohol or drugs influenced their decision to do something sexual.

- Among study participants, 24 to 31 percent reported that they had engaged in more sexual behavior than they had planned to because they had been drinking alcohol or using drugs.
- 12 to 25 percent of study participants reported having unprotected sex because they were drinking alcohol or using drugs.
- More than a quarter of study participants worried about STDs or pregnancy because of something they did sexually while drinking alcohol or using drugs.
- About 1 in 7 study participants said they had used alcohol or drugs to help them feel more comfortable with a sexual partner.

The potential effects of unprotected sex are alarming, especially unplanned pregnancy and STDs. It only takes a single occurrence of unprotected sex for either of these to happen. Early pregnancy can derail a young person's prospects for the normal path of later adulthood, including college, job prospects, and financial independence. An STD can cause embarrassment and humiliation at best or death at worst, such as with the human immunodeficiency virus/acquired immunodeficiency syndrome (HIV/AIDS). The best way for young people to avoid such consequences is to avoid alcohol and sex until they are mature enough to handle them responsibly.

How to Socialize Safely

Tips for staying safe and avoiding sexual assault, especially acts involving alcohol and "date-rape drugs," include:

- Watch your drink at all times. Most "date-rape drugs" have no odor or taste, which makes it easy for someone to spike your drink without your knowledge. If you've left your drink unattended, pour it out.
- Attend social functions with at least one trusted friend (preferably a sober one), who would notice if you were in trouble or acting unusual in some way.
- If you feel drunk but haven't had any alcohol—or if you feel like the effects of your drinking are stronger than usual—find someone who can help you right away.
- Avoid situations where you find yourself alone with someone you don't know very well, especially if one or both of you has been drinking—your ability to make smart choices may be impaired and aggression may be intensified by alcohol.
- Watch for red flags that signal aggressive behavior, including body language or trying to get you into an isolated situation.
- Listen to your gut instincts if you sense trouble in social or sexual situations.
- Don't assume that you're safe just because you're with someone you know.
- If someone is being sexually aggressive, get out of the situation as soon as possible—don't be afraid to be loud or rude.
- Know how alcohol affects you and set limits on how much you drink.

STDs are a potentially devastating consequence of unprotected sex. In the mid-20th century, scientists found that the symptoms of syphilis (which include insanity and death) and other STDs could be controlled with the newly discovered drug penicillin. However, like many antibiotic-controlled diseases, STDs soon became resistant to penicillin, and it now takes even stronger doses to control the symptoms. People who have unprotected sex are at risk for contracting syphilis or any of the following STDs:

- Gonorrhea
- Chlamydia
- Fungal infections
- Human papilloma virus, which causes genital warts and most cases of cervical cancer
- Pelvic inflammatory disease
- Genital herpes
- Bacterial vaginosis
- Human immunodeficiency virus (HIV), which can lead to acquired immune deficiency syndrome (AIDS)
- Pubic lice ("crabs")

Unplanned Sex

When sober, most people are careful in choosing when, where, and who to have sex with. However, the relaxing, brain-numbing effects of alcohol cause many drinkers to lose their inhibitions and have sex with someone they normally wouldn't. Young people who are shy or awkward in social situations may feel bolder and more socially confident when drinking, but the alcohol can give them more than they bargained for, leading to unintended sex. A study conducted by the Harvard University School of Public Health revealed that people who binge drink are even more at risk, with five times the likelihood of having unplanned sex.

As with unprotected sex, unplanned sex carries the same risk of pregnancy and STDs. Many young people who pledge not to have sex outside of a serious relationship or marriage find that their plans for abstinence go awry when they drink alcohol. Avoiding alcohol and its effects on inhibition is one of the best ways to ensure the ability to abstain from sex.

DUAL ADDICTION

People who use alcohol excessively are at risk for becoming dependent on other drugs, including heroin or opiates. The Substance Abuse and Mental Health Services Administration reported that as many as half of all patients admitted to publicly supported alcohol rehab programs had problems with other drugs as well, including pot, crack cocaine, powdered cocaine, methamphetamines (meth), and heroin.

It is not hard to understand why someone would become addicted to more than one substance—the same behaviors and brain chemistry that lead to alcoholism often lead to other forms of dependence. Reasons include:

- The behaviors, lifestyle, and rituals associated with alcohol use are very similar to those of other substances, including nicotine (the primary addictive substance in cigarettes) and cocaine.
- The brain chemistry involved in alcohol addiction is also present in other forms of drug dependence. The opiate receptors are implicated in multiple forms of addiction, playing a role in the euphoric feeling brought on temporarily by drinking or using heroin.
- Psychologically, the factors that lead a person to drink are the same factors that lead to drug use. For example, someone who uses alcohol as a way to escape from problems at home may be just as likely to use drugs for the same reason. Others may combine drugs with alcohol to maximize the intoxicating effects or use one to counteract the effects of the other, such as people who use alcohol to "come down" from a cocaine high.
- When someone has built up a tolerance for alcohol, which makes them more susceptible to addiction (needing more to feel the same effects), they can develop a cross-tolerance, which means they can become tolerant to other drugs, even before using them for the first time. This gives people with cross-tolerance a head start in becoming addicted to the additional substances, meaning an alcoholic may have very little trouble developing a dependence on prescription painkillers.

Researchers at Substance Abuse and Mental Health Services Administration and other organizations who study addiction have found alcohol as well as nicotine to be a common marker for further illicit drug use. This "gateway drug" theory has become more widely accepted because the findings revealed that nearly all teens who use drugs did so only after trying alcohol first.

NUTRITIONAL TROUBLES

A person who drinks too much alcohol may be prone to neglecting their nutritional needs. Alcohol abusers have been known to opt to "drink their lunch" instead of eating a regular meal. Although some alcoholic beverages contain trace amounts of nutrients the body can use, most are simply empty calories that can be a hidden culprit in causing weight gain. For example, a can of beer contains around 150 calories, so having even a couple cans quickly adds useless calories. Drinking causes the body to tell the liver to produce more fat, which also contributes to excess weight. In addition, heavy drinking can also rob the body of essential nutrients, which can lead to weight loss or malnutrition. No two organs are more affected in this way than the liver and pancreas:

- **Liver**—Excessive drinking causes the overworked liver to absorb fewer vitamins, leading to a number of health problems related to vitamin deficiencies, including birth defects (folic acid), vision problems (vitamin A), and weakened bones (vitamin D, which enables calcium absorbance). The liver may also respond to heavy drinking by producing less protein, which can lead to decreased muscle mass.
- **Pancreas**—The two major functions of the pancreas are to aid in digestion and stabilize blood sugar levels. Excessive drinking can impair the pancreas's ability to deliver essential digestive enzymes to the stomach, which leads to poor absorption of nutrients. This can cause neurological problems such as cognitive impairment (thiamine deficiency).

PROBLEMS AT SCHOOL AND WORK

According to a 2002 study conducted by the National Institute on Alcohol Abuse and Alcoholism, college drinking contributes to an estimated 1,400 student deaths and 500,000 injuries. As sobering as that statistic is, there are even more negative aspects of drinking as it relates to students and academic performance. The effects of drinking on students of any age include missed classes, problems concentrating, lower grades, fighting with fellow classmates, falling behind in homework, and dropping out.

Because alcohol's effects are more damaging to the brains of young people under age 25, it can derail many students' academic futures by altering their neurological development, making them less prepared for the demands of high school, college, and careers later in life than their nondrinking peers. Specific brain areas affected include those responsible for verbal skills, learning, memory, and spatial relationships. The idea that alcohol would have a negative effect on school performance seems obvious, and scientific research confirms it:

- The 2000 National Survey on Drug Use and Health revealed lower grade point averages among students aged 12 to 17 who used alcohol compared with their nondrinking peers.
- A study at the University of Washington found that junior high school students who did not use alcohol or drugs received higher scores on the state's reading and math tests than other students.
- In 2001, Columbia University researchers found that high school students who drink are five times more likely to drop out of school than those who do not drink.

- University students who drink are more likely to miss class and fall behind their peers in school.

After high school and college, many drinkers enter the workforce, where they face a whole new set of alcohol-related problems. These include difficulty making it to work on time, inability to concentrate, and hangovers. Excessive drinking and its effects can also cause moodiness and irritability, which makes for a less productive employee and an unpleasant coworker.

6

Alcoholism Today and Beyond

With an abundance of information about alcohol abuse and addiction available, it should be clear that alcoholism is a unique, legitimate disease. Unlike other diseases, alcoholism starts as a behavior that a person engages in willingly and ends up as an impulse that the person loses control over. For that reason, alcoholism is categorized as a psychiatric disorder.

Since the early 1980s, most researchers and addiction professionals have come to consider the behavior of an alcoholic to be not entirely voluntary. The brain of an addict is affected differently by controlled substances like alcohol, compared with the brain of someone who does not have a predisposition for addictive behavior. This helps explain why two people can start out with the same drinking habits but only one becomes addicted.

CHANGING ATTITUDES, TARGETED TREATMENTS

Because of the still-emerging view that alcoholics cannot control their compulsion to drink, alcoholism is slowly being seen less as a moral failing or weakness of character than as a complex blend of physiological, psychological, and genetic factors. This shift in thinking has affected the way addiction professionals, doctors, researchers, and counselors treat alcoholism. This means that the disease is treatable, with options for every step of recovery, from quitting to other rehabilitation to staying sober. Like all addictions, alcoholism is as treatable as chronic medical problems, such as diabetes and high blood pressure.

Treatment options for alcoholism have existed for generations, but the recovery landscape is becoming more sophisticated. From the 1950s through the 1980s, choices for the recovering alcoholic included programs like Alcoholics Anonymous, "drying out" on one's own (with or without formal treatment), jail time, aversion therapy (where the effects of drinking become unpleasant, as with the drug Antabuse), and undergoing religious or psychological scrutiny to examine the so-called lapses in character that lead a person to drink. All of these are still options, some more viable than others.

Over the last few decades, the treatment list now also includes anti-craving drugs, cognitive behavioral therapy, and culturally oriented treatment approaches (why some ethnic or socioeconomic groups may be more likely to become addicted, for example). Treatment advances now focus more on the science of addiction and how tracking changes in the brain of a drinking alcoholic can lead to better medications or therapeutic models.

THE SCIENCE OF ADDICTION

Why does the brain become addicted to alcohol, drugs, gambling, food, and so forth? The rich field of addiction research has yielded many answers to that question, building on the essential ideas of alcohol addiction. In someone with a predisposition for alcohol dependence, drinking affects neurotransmitter activity in the brain more dramatically than in others, although anyone who drinks heavily for a sustained amount of time risks becoming addicted. Brain chemicals that are affected include:

- **Gamma-aminobutyric acid (GABA)**, a neurotransmitter that inhibits the brain's activity to help people sleep, stay calm when overstimulated, and avoid having seizures if they are prone to them (such as people with epilepsy). GABA is also considered a mood-elevating substance that enhances the pleasure a person feels after eating a good meal, having sex, or drinking a glass of wine.
- **Serotonin**, another mood-elevating neurotransmitter whose activity can be increased after heavy or sustained drinking. Serotonin is a chemical messenger that influences mood, appetite, sleep, sex drive, and memory. Alcohol not only increases the effects of serotonin but affects serotonin receptors, which play a role in the brain's reward system, intoxication, and withdrawal symptoms.
- **Glutamate**, an amino acid, otherwise known as a building block for protein in the body, that is also a neurotransmitter that plays a big role in memory and learning. In contrast to GABA, glutamate is an excitatory chemical

that can cause psychosis and seizures if the body produces too much. Drinking too much alcohol causes the body to produce less glutamate, while increasing the brain's sensitivity to it. Eventually, the brain of a heavy drinker will try to make more dampening chemicals like GABA to counteract the increased sensitivity to glutamate.

- **Dopamine**, a neurotransmitter associated with concentration, mood, learning, and, most importantly to alcoholics, reward. In other words, alcohol (as well as nicotine and other drugs) triggers an increase in dopamine production, leading to the euphoric feeling people get when they're tipsy or intoxicated. For this reason, dopamine is a primary means for the brain's pleasure center to be "hijacked" by alcohol and become less responsive to non-alcohol-related experiences.

In people who are not alcoholics, the brain regulates the production, sensitivity, and release of these chemicals. After a person has experienced the chemicals' pleasurable effects, comparable to the intoxication of drinking or taking drugs, the body must then normalize its chemistry and bring itself back in balance. It does this by releasing counterbalancing hormones, such as stress hormones, and lowering the amount of other sedating or pleasurable chemicals, bringing the brain back to equilibrium.

Among heavy or steady drinkers, however, the brain often doesn't have time to return the body to this state of equilibrium before the next wave of intoxication disrupts the balance. If this happens, the brain adjusts to the increased neurotransmitter activity and starts requiring more of the alcohol-triggered chemicals for the body to feel "normal." In other words, the more a person drinks, the more he or she needs to drink in order to feel calm. This is what is known as tolerance, and the higher a person's tolerance for alcohol the more likely he or she is to become addicted.

If a person develops too high a tolerance for alcohol, he or she will eventually stop feeling the pleasurable effects of drinking and will instead need to use alcohol to stave off the uncomfortable, or even scary, effects of stopping. At this stage, without alcohol a person becomes moody, anxious, depressed, or irritable until he or she can find a drink. He or she may even experience withdrawal symptoms, such as trembling and nausea. Such symptoms are a marker of physiological dependence. This is often the point at which addiction has set in. Researchers are not sure if this is a permanent state or a reversible one—many drinkers who have been sober for years are still haunted by cravings, which is why relapse is a common pitfall for recovering alcoholics.

Such cravings are at the core of many clinical studies on alcoholism treatment today. These findings have brought scientists and everyday people alike a long way toward seeing a more truthful view of the alcoholic than one of weak character or lack of self-control. Neurological evidence of cravings does not absolve drinkers from their behaviors related to alcohol, but it does help explain why most alcoholics cannot control their behavior or quit without help. Several anti-craving drugs and therapies as well as other alcoholism treatment options have already been developed, with more to come.

NEW MEDICATIONS

The use of drug-based treatments for alcoholism mostly focuses on medications as a supplement to other options, including counseling and 12-step groups. Medications aren't seen as a suitable treatment by themselves, but as tools to help addiction professionals keep alcoholics from relapsing. These drugs have proven to be a useful weapon in the fight against alcoholism relapse and are generally underused. In addition to naltrexone (an anti-craving medication) and the decades-old aversion drug disulfiram, another anti-craving drug called acamprosate was introduced in 2004. Medical researchers aren't slowing down in the quest to modify existing medications and discover new drug treatments for alcoholics.

New Form of Naltrexone

Naltrexone is an opioid antagonist that helps curb alcohol cravings by inhibiting the pleasure centers normally stimulated by drinking. While this provides some relief for drinkers in recovery, researchers in San Francisco may have extracted an even more effective version of the drug by creating a new form of naltrexone called SoRI-9409.

The SoRI-9409 compound appears to provide stronger anti-craving benefits than those of naltrexone's original formulation, and with fewer side effects. Furthermore, the alcohol-addicted lab rats that were the subjects of the San Francisco study did not start drinking heavily again in the month following their removal from the drug. This feature, should it test well in humans also, would make SoRI-9409 an exciting long-term treatment option because there wouldn't be as high a chance of relapse after a person stopped taking the drug.

Ondansetron

The drug ondansetron is most commonly known to doctors as a treatment for the nausea and vomiting that often occur in people undergoing chemotherapy. However, ondansetron may also prove to be a promising new treatment for alcohol addiction as well.

As with many such findings, ondansetron's effects on alcohol consumption were discovered by accident when researchers at the University of Texas noticed that people taking the drug for non-alcohol-related reasons reported a reduced urge to drink. After ruling out other factors for quitting alcohol, the researchers determined that it was probably ondansetron's change of the pleasurable effects of serotonin that lead to the reduction of drinking.

Ondansetron has been found to be more effective in treating early-onset alcoholics (those who become addicted before the age of 25) than in their older counterparts. Since these addicts tend to resist other forms of treatment, have antisocial behaviors, and a family history of alcoholism, they are often challenging to treat. That makes the discovery of ondansetron's anti-craving properties for early-onset alcoholics even more encouraging.

Since nausea and anxiety can occur in people who are trying to quit drinking, ondansetron is doubly effective for addressing these symptoms. The University of Texas researchers also found a potent treatment for alcohol cravings by combining ondansetron with the anti-craving drugs naltrexone and acamprosate.

Varenicline

Smokers have had the drug varenicline available since 2007 to help them stave off cigarette cravings. The drug works by preventing nicotine from triggering the release of dopamine, a brain chemical that is part of the pleasurable sensation smokers experience from cigarettes. A recent study found that varenicline also helps curb cravings in nicotine-addicted laboratory rats, and there is much anecdotal evidence from people who tried the drug to quit smoking and then found that it also helped them drink less.

Rats given the drug were found to cut their drinking in half. Almost as important, the rats who were taken off the drug did not engage in the sort of "rebound" binge-drinking that has been a discouraging hallmark of other treatments. This is an important signal that the drug is decreasing the reward system that causes people to become addicted to alcohol. Researchers think the drug works by affecting the alcohol-activated receptors of the brain.

A prime advantage of varenicline is that it is proving to be safe and effective without the side effects of other alcohol treatment medications, although its own side effects are still being evaluated. It is also not metabolized by the liver, which makes it twice as beneficial to heavy drinkers with compromised liver function. Since smoking and drinking are often coexisting behaviors and addictions, varenicline prevents cravings for two substances at once. Clinical trials on humans will prove to be the drug's final test, but these early results are intriguing.

NON-DRUG APPROACHES

A number of non-drug options are emerging to help people with alcohol dependence fight the addiction. New therapies like these are often most intriguing to alcoholics because they do not involve yet another drug or substance, something that can perhaps help support the mindset of "coming clean." New nondrug treatment approaches include deep brain stimulation and motivational enhancement therapy.

Deep Brain Stimulation

Most often associated with treatment of movement disorders like Parkinson's disease, deep brain stimulation (DBS) involves a series of electrodes inserted into the brain to stimulate areas that normally could not be accessed without invasive surgery. The electrical pulse delivered to the brain by a DBS device can manipulate parts of the brain that have been damaged by age or trauma into functioning normally again. DBS has shown promise for Parkinson's disease and other disorders, such as epilepsy and depression. It may also be a future treatment for alcohol addiction, as evidenced by an accidental discovery by German researchers.

In October 2007, the *Journal of Neurology, Neurosurgery, and Psychiatry* reported that German physicians stumbled across a potentially therapeutic use of DBS for treating alcohol dependence. The researchers, hoping to cure an alcoholic of depression and anxiety by using DBS, were surprised to find that the treatment instead caused him to quit drinking (the symptoms of depression persisted). The DBS targeted an area of the brain called the nucleus accumbens, which regulates the reward system that is associated with addiction—in other words, the part of the brain that causes cravings. How it was able to dampen the cravings is still not clear. More research is needed to build on this discovery, such as:

- If another team of researchers could duplicate the results with larger numbers of people.
- How frequently DBS treatments would be needed to help drinkers avoid relapse.
- How long DBS treatments would be needed after a drinker quits in order to prevent relapse.
- If DBS's anti-craving effects would last indefinitely or if it would wear off after a certain amount of time.

More studies of this therapy are underway for other forms of addiction besides alcoholism. The August 2008 edition of *The Journal of Neuroscience* published study results from a team of researchers evaluating the use of DBS in treating cocaine addicts, who have a notoriously high rate of relapse. The study showed that DBS stimulation could be a "potential therapeutic option in the treatment of severe cocaine addiction" by reducing cravings in cocaine-addicted lab rats.

If DBS does turn out to be a viable treatment for addiction, one of its principle benefits could be that someone receiving it might be able to avoid the potential side effects of anti-craving drugs. Of course, the potential side effects of DBS would have to be weighed as well, but this treatment seems to show great promise for problem drinkers. It may also provide an alternative or supplement for people whose cravings have not responded to other treatments.

Motivational Enhancement Therapy

Motivational enhancement therapy (MET) is not a new treatment for alcoholism and other addictions, but it is relatively recent. MET is a 6-step process:

- The first stage is precontemplation. Precontemplators are not considering a change and are unaware or unwilling to admit that a problem exists.
- Once aware of the problem, precontemplators can move into the contemplation stage. If someone is truly self-medicating with alcohol, there is usually not much difficulty moving him or her into this stage. Contemplators are ambivalent about change. While they may not be considering it immediately, they are aware of the effects of drinking on their lives. Drinkers may get stuck in this stage if they are worried about symptoms like anxiety if they stop drinking.
- The third stage is preparation or determination. A drinker in this stage is making a commitment to take action and developing a strategy for change. Remember that most drinkers do not actually know how to change. Some may need several sessions of MET to prepare for the change, but eventually most will reach the conclusion that they'll feel better without alcohol. In this stage, the drinker may start considering options such as Alcoholics Anonymous or other self-help groups and outpatient substance abuse treatment programs.
- The fourth stage is action, which involves implementing the plan and practicing being sober for three to six months.
- Action is followed by maintenance, the stage where a person's newfound sobriety is sustained for an extended period of time (up to five years) and is part of everyday life.
- The final stage, relapse, is not inevitable, but it is common for many addicts. A relapse must be viewed as a learning experience and a time for re-evaluation of the treatment plan by a counselor or other provider. If a drinker is unable to stop abusing alcohol, he or she may need detoxification, medications for anxiety, or some type of psychotherapy.

The stages of change occur in sequence, but a relapse can place a person back to any previous stage. The length of time spent in any one stage can vary from brief to a lifetime.

Unlike other forms of counseling, which rely heavily on a therapist's expertise and direction, MET uses a person's own resources for realizing change from within. As the name would suggest, during MET a therapist's responsibility is to build a sense of motivation that is intrinsic. This helps a drinker see for himself or herself the reasons for quitting and become inspired to act on those reasons without having to be forced to do so by his or her family, a supervisor at work, or a court order.

An advantage of MET is that it does not exclude other effective forms of counseling, such as cognitive behavioral therapy or 12-step therapy. In fact, MET has sometimes been shown to be more effective when combined with one or both of these other treatments.

ALCOHOLISM AND MODERN RESEARCH

The research of alcoholism treatment options and its resulting advances owes a lot to innovative thinking on the part of scientists and addiction professionals, but there is another factor that has contributed to the improved outlook for alcoholism: improved research methods. While using clinical methods for treating alcoholics is not especially new, researchers have done more in the last 25 years to measure and validate the success of various treatment options. A healthcare provider treating alcoholism or another type of addiction now can be reassured that the medication or therapy has likely been tested on a control group in a clinical trial, whereas before doctors might simply rely on their judgment and anecdotal evidence to choose a treatment option and hope for the best.

In addition to giving doctors this peace of mind, another important outcome of more rigorous research methods is that they have led to improvements through combining certain treatments. For example, the 12-step programs pioneered by Alcoholics Anonymous (AA), in which the drinker follows a series of steps that provide guidance and structure during recovery, seemed to be helping people quit drinking, but until the 1990s AA's methods had not been extensively studied to see why or even if they succeeded.

Several studies in the 1990s helped shed some light on AA's success, with one revealing that 12-step programs work better when combined with inpatient treatment programs and counseling. It is common to think that the more treatment a person gets the more likely he or she is to succeed, but such results do provide clinicians and counselors with a means to give alcoholics more targeted treatment. Another study found that 12-step programs are more effective for helping drinkers achieve long-term abstinence and the ability to keep a job after quitting drinking than those who had been treated with cognitive behavioral therapy alone.

REMOVING BARRIERS: ALCOHOLISM TREATMENT AND INSURANCE

Because of changing perceptions of alcoholism and addiction, the still-evolving idea that substance abuse is caused by a complex blend of physiological, genetic, and psychological factors that put the problem beyond users' control, people addicted to alcohol have benefited in another way: access to care. Because alcoholism was not considered a legitimate disease until relatively recently, it could not be treated medically as a disease. Even doctors who may have bought into the disease theory of alcoholism early on were in the minority and had few options for treating it. There was little in the way of research and development, government funding, or mainstream efforts to assign cause or cure. Fortunately, a handful of forward-thinking scientists and researchers, and their legions of advocates who championed such ideas, were able to advance what finally came to be known as the disease theory of alcoholism.

The Disease Theory of Alcoholism: A Brief History

The disease theory has its origins in the late 18th century and early 19th century, a time of accelerated medical and scientific advancements that included early forms of surgery, the first successful blood transfusion, and the publication of Darwin's *The Origin of Species*. It was in this intellectually fertile environment that some physicians started considering how alcohol affected the human body. Before this idea, alcohol was thought of as a safe alternative to water in many cities, as well as a perfectly acceptable painkiller, mood elevator, and general tonic for a variety of ills. People who drank too much were considered morally unfit or weak and were usually punished, shunned, or looked down upon. Leading scientists knew at least that drinking too much could lead to mental illness and social mayhem on a large scale.

One of the earliest acknowledged proponents of the disease theory of alcoholism was a British physician named Thomas Trotter. Working with the mentally ill in the rapidly expanding insane asylums of the Victorian era, Dr. Trotter began to notice that heavy drinking was more likely to be the cause of debauched, immoral tendencies and behavior, and not necessarily the other way around. In other words, the drinker was sick, could not control himself or herself, and suffered from mental illness as a result of prolonged heavy drinking. Dr. Trotter saw this as a physiological problem and referred to these probable alcoholics as "inebriates" who had no choice in their behavior. His contemporary, another important pioneer of the disease theory of alcoholism, Dr. C. von Brühl-Cramer, coined the term "dipsomania" to describe his own early observations on alcoholism. In his most famous work, "An Essay, Medical, Philosophical, and Chemical, on Drunkenness and Its Effects on the Human Body" published in 1813, Dr. Trotter described the compromised, intoxicated brain of an otherwise sensible man in simple terms: "The man is now drunk, and whatever he says or does betrays the errors of the thinking principle." Thus, while many scientists would build on Dr. Trotter's initial discoveries, he was the first researcher to call for removing alcohol treatment from the hands of "parsons and moralists," who tended to see excessive drinking as a punishable offense, and make it the work of the scientific community, who viewed addiction as a rational problem to be solved and not condemned as mere vice. It is hard to imagine today, but at the time Dr. Trotter's observations were considered radical and groundbreaking, leading to a more compassionate and science-based view of excessive drinking.

Meanwhile across the Atlantic, a Philadelphia physician named Benjamin Rush, one of Trotter's fellow alumni from Edinburgh College of Medicine in Scotland, was arriving at some similar conclusions on the origins of excessive drinking. Dr. Rush, famously known as the father of American psychiatry, was one of the first physicians to accurately identify the health hazards associated with excessive drinking. In his role as surgeon general of the Continental army during the American Revolution, Dr. Rush observed the alcohol-related behavior of the soldiers around him. He noticed that drinking started out as a voluntary behavior that became involuntary in certain men. He identified this problem as a loss of willpower that left the drinker helpless to quit. Dr. Rush had signed the Declaration of Independence, counseled U.S. presidents, and established himself as an eminent doctor, humanitarian, and educator—he was very well known in American life. Thus, his discoveries were very influential in advancing the idea that alcohol dependence was not a vice, but rather a medical—and specifically psychiatric—condition. Both Dr. Trotter and Dr. Rush were unique in being among the first physicians studying addiction to advocate total abstinence from alcohol. The former envisioned physical factors playing a key role in addiction, while the latter focused on drinking as a mental health issue.

As the rationalist influence of scientists like Dr. Trotter, Dr. Brühl-Cramer, and Dr. Rush spread throughout the late 19th century and early 20th century, many of their peers in the research community developed a more clinical, compassionate, and less moralistic view of alcoholism. This led to such measures as physician-operated "inebriate asylums," which slowly but steadily grew in number by the early 1900s, as well as the roots of the prohibition movement in the United States during the early 20th century. However, among most members of the public, whose perceptions were more influenced by the strict societal norms of the 19th century that governed behavior like drinking, the idea of alcoholism as a vice and moral weakness persisted. It was not until the mid-20th century that the disease theory of alcoholism started gaining more widespread and public acceptance. This was likely due in large part to the founding of Alcoholics Anonymous in the 1930s, as well as the pioneering work of an American physician named E. Morton Jellinek.

Jellinek and a Framework for Defining Alcoholism

While many scientists and doctors had defined or accepted alcoholism as a disease by the mid-20th century, Dr. E.M. Jellinek was the first to coin the phrase "disease concept of alcoholism," which was also the name of his most famous book, published in 1960. Dr. Jellinek furthered and accelerated the notion of alcohol addiction as a legitimate disorder, and it was his research that influenced such policy-related moves as the American Medical Association's designation of alcohol as an illness and not a character flaw in 1956, as well as similar declarations by the World Health Organization and the American Psychiatric Association.

Dr. Jellinek was the first scientist to create classifications for alcoholism, based on the progression of the disease and identifiable types of alcoholics. He identified alcoholism as a progressive disorder, with stages of addiction that intensify as the person's tolerance to alcohol's effects increases. The four progressive phases are as follows:

- **Pre-alcoholic phase:** In this phase, the drinker's alcohol consumption starts out as a social or recreational activity, gradually becoming a way for the person to relax, unwind, and deal with stress. At this stage, this drinker may seem fine, with drinking habits that are indistinguishable from those of his or her peers.
- **Prodromal phase:** At this point, the drinker has identified alcohol as an essential means for escaping life's problems and will seek out reasons to drink. The person may have his or her drinking habit under control, but will fall into a pattern of alcohol abuse that includes drinking to get drunk, becoming reckless while drinking, blacking out (experiencing temporary memory loss, not to be confused with passing out) and forgetting events and occurrences that happened during a bout of drinking, using alcohol in secret and gulping drinks when no one is looking, furtively spiking nonalcoholic drinks, and experiencing more frequent and severe hangovers than before.
- **Crucial phase:** The most obvious change that gets the alcoholic to this stage is loss of control, which signals that physical addiction has set in. Accordingly, the person's drinking habit will become more conspicuous to others, as getting alcohol becomes more important than hiding the need for it. Signs of the crucial phase of alcoholism include drinking alone or with other alcoholics, drinking with people outside of the normal social circle because of a shared feeling that only other heavy drinkers can understand each other, drinking upon waking up in the morning, failed attempts at quitting, making excuses to drink or rationalizing their habits ("I needed a drink to deal with a bad day at work"), and needing medical care for health-related problems of heavy drinking (although offering no admission

of a drinking problem). In this phase, the drinker's relationships with family, friends, coworkers, and supervisors become strained and his or her loved ones may start avoiding them. The person has started making alcohol a priority over all other activities and relationships.

- **Critical phase:** Until the critical phase, the alcoholic may have had a choice whether to drink or not—at least before he or she started the first drink of the day. But now, the drinker has lost all power over that choice and must drink to avoid the terrifying aspect of withdrawal symptoms. If the problem hasn't been obvious up to this point, it will be now, because the person will show clear signs of excessive drinking. If not able to find a drink, the critical-phase alcoholic may tremble, sweat profusely, and experience hallucinations—all of which comprise the condition known as delirium tremens, a potentially life-threatening condition. Fear of these symptoms drives the person to always have alcohol nearby, sometimes hidden in different parts of the house, in the car, or in a flask carried in a pocket. The person may go on prolonged bouts of drinking, losing all pretense of caring about relationships, eating, keeping a job, or even needing shelter. At this point, the drinking's toll on the brain leads to anxiety, paranoia, and even hostility or violence. This is the phase at which the drinker is most likely to admit defeat and concede utter lack of control over alcohol, particularly if he or she is suffering from a health problem related to long-term heavy drinking, such as alcoholic psychosis, coma, or cirrhosis. If the person isn't admitting to a problem at this stage, he or she is likely to succumb to their habit unless physically forced to quit.

In addition to these four progressive phases, Dr. Jellinek, in his studies of heavy drinkers around the world, formulated a list of several types of alcoholics, as opposed to degree of addiction. Each category is named by a letter in the Greek alphabet:

- **Alpha alcoholism:** This type of drinker has a psychological addiction to alcohol but hasn't lost control of his or her drinking. The alpha alcoholic uses drinking as a way to deal with every day stresses and pressures of life. Some observers may call this type of alcoholic a problem drinker, and the person's alcohol use may jeopardize his or her home life, job, and relationships. This kind of drinker won't necessarily progress to a more advanced stage of drinking, although it's possible.
- **Beta alcoholism:** A beta alcoholic may suffer physical health problems, such as liver failure or inflammation of the stomach lining, from heavy drinking. However, the person has not yet developed a dependence. This paradoxical situation, in Dr. Jellinek's observations, is more likely to occur in cultures where heavy drinking is common but where people don't have adequate access to good nutrition.

- **Gamma alcoholism**: Dr. Jellinek observed that this was the most common type of alcoholic he studied, especially in the United States and among members of AA. The psychological dependence has become physiological in this category of alcoholic, and the person's drinking is by now disrupting his or her relationships. Typically, this type of heavy drinker has probably lost control of his or her alcohol consumption and may start showing signs of physical withdrawal upon trying to quit.
- **Delta alcoholism**: Like the gamma alcoholic, this type of drinker is physiologically and psychologically dependent. However, unlike the gamma alcoholic, the delta alcoholic hasn't lost complete control of his or her drinking. He or she will suffer withdrawal symptoms after a day or so of no drinking, but can get through a social occasion or other short periods of time without drinking to excess.
- **Epsilon alcoholism**: This stand-alone category of heavy drinking represents what Dr. Jellinek called "periodic alcoholism." This type of alcoholic is identifiable by regular bouts of binge-drinking, but Dr. Jellinek didn't study this type enough to elaborate beyond that.

After deriving these classifications of alcoholic types, Dr. Jellinek stated that not every species of heavy drinker was someone with a disease. Critics of Dr. Jellinek's work point out that he often failed to identify the difference between a problem drinker (or alcoholic) and someone who drank heavily but within normal limits. This is often a blurry line for many people trying to navigate the complexities of a heavy drinker's behavioral patterns. When does habitual heavy drinking turn into a disease? And is someone with a psychological dependence on alcohol in the same need of treatment as a person with physical withdrawal symptoms? Dr. Jellinek's work was groundbreaking and highly influential, but it didn't eliminate the controversy over the disease theory of alcoholism.

In fact, despite the work of Dr. Trotter, Dr. Rush, and Dr. Jellinek, the idea of alcoholism as a chronic disease remains the subject of much debate. Dr. Jellinek himself noted that the controversy arose from too many definitions of alcoholism and not enough definitions of disease. Indeed, most professionals who have accepted the disease theory of alcoholism have done so by expanding the idea of disease to include the involuntary nature of alcoholism.

One of the most notable and vocal critics of the idea is psychologist Stanton Peele, a best-selling author on the subject of addiction who dismisses the disease theory as a means for alcoholics to be absolved of personal responsibility for their actions. In addition, Dr. Peele argues that the disease theory was too easily accepted into the mainstream medical community, probably because it dovetailed so handily with the very influential ideas of AA, which were as enormously popular in Dr. Jellinek's time as they are now. Furthermore, Dr. Peele and other critics argue that abstinence is not the only solution to addiction and that, when properly counseled, people with a drinking problem can be cured of their dependence and safely return to moderate consumption of alcohol. Dr. Peele also notes that the popularity and success of the disease theory of alcoholism has led to the medicalization of other everyday ills, including premenstrual tension, gambling, overeating, child abuse, and even shopping.

Dr. Peele's fellow critic Herbert Fingarette also shares this notion, arguing that, among other problems, designating an alcoholic as someone with a disease affords that person with "special benefits, in employment, health, and civil rights law, provided they can prove that their drinking is persistent and very heavy." In other words, people identified as alcoholics get away with more because their behavior is seen as involuntary. He goes on to call the disease concept a "useful lie" upon which scores of treatment centers and addictions professionals have profited, especially as insurance companies have started covering addiction disorders more thoroughly. Fingarette and Dr. Peele see alcohol addiction as a human, psychological, and social issue, not a medical one.

These criticisms are important in the bigger discussion of alcoholism as a disease, and scientists may never fully figure out what the true culprit is in the development of addiction. It's up to each individual to formulate his or her own opinion, because no one institution has conclusively proved their position on the disease concept, and there are valid points on each side.

One aspect of the debate that may be helpful is to consider the continuously evolving diagnostic criteria for several major medical groups, because those criteria have come to occupy an important place in the alcohol treatment landscape.

Naming the Unnamable: Diagnosing Alcoholism

Because of the advances in thinking that emerged from Dr. Jellinek's research and the rising prominence of the ideas of AA, several medical associations fell in line with the disease concept of alcoholism, as we have already seen. These groups included the American Medical Association (AMA) and the American Psychiatric Association (APA), two of the most powerful guideline-setting organizations in the medical field. Of course, neither of these were the first to set forth such criteria—the National Institute on Alcohol Abuse and Alcoholism (NIAAA) reports that at least 39 such sets of diagnostic criteria existed before 1940. Dr. Jellinek's Greek-lettered list of alcoholism types could be considered another pioneering work of addiction diagnosis.

Why is it so important for physicians and their alcohol-addicted patients to work with these lists? For one thing, it allows doctors to work with a set of consistent rules that determine which behaviors or symptoms are evidence of a certain disease or condition. In other words, since a variety of researchers have arrived at these criteria, the physician knows he or she does not have to duplicate this work, and that the criteria are trustworthy.

More importantly for many alcoholics is that diagnostic criteria enable them to receive critically important treatment for their addiction. Or as summarized by the NIAAA, "the criteria help healthcare insurers to decide whether treatment will be reimbursed; and allow patients access to medical insurance coverage" (1995).

In 1956, when the AMA identified alcoholism as a disease, it did so because alcohol dependence met five requirements for such a designation: it had a pattern of symptoms, it's a chronic disorder, the symptoms progress, there's a risk of relapse, and it's treatable.

As for the APA, it defines alcohol addiction as indicated by these factors (excerpted from the *Diagnostic & Statistical Manual of Mental Disorders*, Fourth Edition, text revised):

- Physiological dependence on alcohol is indicated by evidence of tolerance or symptoms of withdrawal. Especially if associated with a history of withdrawal, physiological dependence is an indication of a more severe clinical course overall (i.e., earlier onset, higher levels of intake, more alcohol-related problems).
- Alcohol withdrawal is characterized by symptoms that develop 4–12 hours or so after the reduction of intake following prolonged, heavy, alcohol ingestion. Because withdrawal from alcohol can be unpleasant and intense, individuals with alcohol dependence may continue to consume alcohol, despite adverse consequences, often to avoid or to relieve the symptoms of withdrawal.
- Once a pattern of compulsive use develops, individuals with dependence may devote substantial periods of time to obtaining and consuming alcoholic beverages. These individuals often continue to use alcohol despite evidence of adverse psychological or physical consequences (e.g., depression, blackouts, liver disease, or other sequelae).

In other words, the drinker suffers physical withdrawal symptoms, those symptoms develop within hours of quitting, drinkers keep drinking to avoid the symptoms, and the addicted drinker will keep using alcohol despite any the problems it may cause to his or her mental and physical health.

Both the AMA and APA diagnostic criteria are straightforward enough for even a layperson to understand, so it's hard to imagine a time when they didn't exist. Because of such criteria, the diagnosis of alcohol addiction is easier to define for advocates of health insurance reform, which has gradually led to better coverage for alcohols in need of treatment.

Alcoholism and Health Insurance Parity

Today, alcoholism is the "disease" instead of the "weakness of character." Even though there are plenty of critics of this notion, for the most part the majority of doctors and other healthcare practitioners believe that alcohol dependence is a chronic disease just like diabetes or lupus. And just like with other chronic diseases, alcoholism treatment is constantly evolving, with advocates and patient groups making a case to get public and private research funds for continued study and incremental improvements to the current treatment tools. As a result, now doctors in the U.S., for example, have not one but two anti-craving drugs (naltrexone and acamprosate) that weren't available two decades ago.

In addition to the advances in alcoholism science and research that have brought about such medications, being able to quantify addiction through diagnostic criteria is yielding another outcome: health insurance parity. In the last few decades, lingering doubts regarding the validity of alcoholism as a disease have made it difficult for alcoholics to get their treatment costs covered by health insurance. This problem isn't unique to alcoholics—health insurance parity is an issue faced by many groups, including those with autism and people with mood disorders. Those advocating for the coverage of substance abuse treatment have usually worked in partnership with those in the mental health community seeking the same insurance benefits.

The Story of Health Insurance Parity

What does health insurance parity mean? Simply put, that substance abuse and mental health conditions should be covered in the same way as medical or surgical conditions. In the 1970s and 1980s, as healthcare costs rose sharply, most insurers tightened rules on what conditions they would cover—most wouldn't pay for treatment for addiction-related conditions at all. Those that would offered only limited coverage. Understandably, proponents of substance abuse and mental health treatment saw this as a form of discrimination and undertook political and social measures to correct the imbalance in coverage. These advocates included members of the U.S. Congress, such as late Minnesota senator Paul Wellstone and Rhode Island representative Patrick Kennedy, as well as doctors, scientists and other researchers, substance abuse professionals, recovering addicts, authors, and everyday champions for people suffering from addiction and mental health disorders. Even with changing attitudes about the involuntary nature of alcoholism, insurance companies were reluctant to provide the same coverage as for medical and surgical disorders. Critics of this lack of parity likened it to insurance companies refusing equal coverage for people with other chronic disorders, such as high blood pressure or diabetes.

Some progress was made in the 1980s, but there were still inequalities. For example, even if addiction treatment was covered, insurance companies would put a cap on the number of treatments people could receive, with monetary limits that made it impossible for some to afford even partially covered treatment. Opponents of these policies argued that addiction is a complex brain-linked condition requiring more than a one-time treatment—in most cases, heavy drinkers and drug users need long-term follow-up counseling, life-skills training, and other adjuncts of their core treatment to ensure successful attempts at sobriety. Furthermore, since a common component of alcohol recovery is relapse, a single treatment wouldn't suffice for many addicts who need more than one attempt at quitting.

Another insurance-related obstacle during the 1980s was the rise of the managed-care model of health insurance, a cost-conscious system in which a primary care physician is designated as a sort of gatekeeper in deciding whether a patient can receive specialty medical care, such as substance abuse treatment. Managed care insurance rules often meant that an alcoholic or addict would only receive treatment if his or her primary care physician deemed it necessary. Alcoholics and other addicts were unable to seek this treatment on their own without insurance-mandated clearance from their doctor. Doctors who didn't view alcoholism as a disease were unlikely to recommend the treatment. Advocates for alcoholism treatment felt that addicts had to jump through bureaucratic hoops and subject themselves to a primary care physician's whims to get treatment under the managed care system.

For their part, insurance companies strongly resisted attempts to provide equal coverage for mental health and substance-abuse treatment, largely because of fears of the high cost of treatment. There were also doubts about the effectiveness of treatment, due no doubt to a lack of understanding on the process of addiction treatment. For example, some observers might view relapse as a failure of treatment rather than a common setback that doesn't necessarily signal that the treatment isn't working. Despite continued activism, insurers continued to impose stricter spending caps, higher deductibles, and higher co-payments for mental health and substance-abuse treatments.

While many U.S. states enacted parity laws for mental health and substance-abuse insurance coverage, there were no significant protections at the federal level until 1996, when Congress passed the Mental Health Parity Act (MHPA), which featured two important provisions:

- Parity of mental health benefits with medical and surgical benefits with respect to the application of aggregate lifetime and annual dollar limits under a group health plan
- A requirement that employers retain discretion regarding the extent and scope of mental health benefits offered to workers and their families (including cost sharing, limits on numbers of visits or days of coverage, and requirements relating to medical necessity)

The law advanced the goals of the mental health community somewhat, but it didn't prevent insurance companies from circumventing the spirit of the law by putting measures in place such as limiting the number of treatment sessions needed by someone seeking care, and it didn't require insurers to cover mental health conditions at all. Some states responded to these perceived inadequacies of the MHPA by enacting even stronger parity laws at the state level, but this still didn't guarantee equal coverage on a consistent basis. It only meant that a person's likelihood of receiving insurance coverage was determined by where he or she lived, not by his or her actual needs. Most importantly for sufferers of addiction and their advocates, there were no provisions in the MHPA for substance abuse treatment.

With the encouraging but incomplete victory of the MHPA, advocates pressed on and more substance-abuse-related organizations like the American Society of Addiction Medicine (ASAM) and the American Managed Behavioral Healthcare Association (AMBHA) issuing statements like this one in support of insurance parity:

> Benefit plans for the treatment of addictive disorders, in both the public and private sectors, shall be comprehensive; i.e., they shall cover the entire continuum of clinically effective and appropriate services provided by competent licensed professionals, and should provide identical coverage and funding to those benefits covering physical illness, with the same provisions, lifetime benefits, and catastrophic coverage.

In the last decade of the 20th century and into the new millennium, study after study continued to pile on evidence that not only was alcoholism a legitimate and chronic illness, but it was one of heavy social costs and not just medical costs. The admittedly high, up-front investment of treating people with substance abuse is likely to be a fraction of the cost of untreated alcoholism. Lost productivity at work, crime, and fractured families would probably exact a larger financial and social toll than the cost of treatment, in the view of insurance-parity supporters. As outlined by ASAM fellow and board member Dr. Ken Roy, these are the logical steps and reasons why insurance parity is so vitally important:

1. Health insurance provides financial coverage for diagnosis, treatment, and prevention of acute and chronic diseases.
2. Addiction medicine is involved in the diagnosis, treatment, and prevention of substance related disorders, which are acute or chronic diseases.
3. Addiction is a complex neurobehavioral disorder, involving biochemical abnormalities of the brain that involve reinforcement and reward systems of the central nervous system; addiction is manifested by aberrant behaviors that can compulsively persist despite adverse consequences from those behaviors; addiction is not a character weakness.

4. Addiction diagnosis is objective, standardized, and scientific, no less so than for other chronic diseases.
5. Addiction treatment is effective.
6. Barriers to the effectiveness of addiction treatment are the same as barriers to the effectiveness of treatment interventions for other chronic diseases: patient compliance and readiness to change, socioeconomic complications to care, delivery and management, and comorbid emotional-behavioral conditions all adversely impact treatment success for substance addiction and for other chronic illnesses. There is nothing intrinsic to addiction treatment that should generate pessimism about treatment efficacy rates, and such pessimism is not supported by clinical research or experience.
7. Relapse is inherent in addictive disease, but also inherent in virtually all chronic disease; relapse is usually a sign of chronicity, not a sign of treatment failure. By relapse, we mean a return to the signs and symptoms meeting criteria for a substance use disorder, not a return to use per se.
8. Insurance benefits for addiction treatment should be equivalent to benefits for the treatment of other chronic diseases.
9. Treatment for the disease of addiction is cost-effective, and can be cost-saving for the healthcare system overall.
10. Because of medical cost offsets, to NOT treat the disease of addiction is costly, economically as well as socially; benefit structures should not create barriers to effective intervention to diagnose and treat addiction.

Goals of insurance-parity activists included increasing the consistency among states, whose various parity laws contained wildly differing rules. Another goal was to achieve consensus on how to include addiction and alcoholism in the definition of disease, and what it means for a health-related service to be considered medically or clinically necessary. Parity supporters encouraged a national dialogue among politicians, consumers, families of addicts, employers, managed care organizations, and state and federal governments.

The Mental Health Parity and Addiction Equity Act of 2008

In October of 2008, the considerable efforts of activists paid off in a big way with the passage of the Mental Health Parity and Addiction Equity Act of 2008 (MHPAEA), which was quickly added as an attachment to a bailout bill intended to stimulate the nation's severely sagging economy. The newly shifting political winds had installed a democratic U.S. president and Congress, and with democrats being traditional allies of inclusiveness and universal coverage in healthcare, insurance companies finally gave in, and most supported the bill and the parity it brought.

The law corrected many of the perceived inadequacies of the 12-year-old MHPA. For example, although the law does not require insurance companies to cover conditions related to mental health and substance abuse, it does require those conditions, when included in a health insurance policy, to be covered at the same level as medical and surgical conditions. It also requires that plans offering out-of-network benefits (out-of-network providers are those that haven't signed an agreement with the insurance company to provide services at an agreed-upon cost structure) for medical and surgical conditions to offer those out-of-network benefits for mental health and addiction treatment as well.

The passage of the MHPAEA means that many people suffering from alcoholism are certain to have increased access to the care and treatment they need. Insurers will no longer be allowed to put a cap on the number of covered days for inpatient rehab treatment or limit how many outpatient visits the addict may need for follow-up treatment. The mental health aspect of the law will also provide indirect benefits to those suffering from addictions disorders as well, because they will receive more thorough treatment for the disorders that can lead to drinking, such as anxiety and depression, which also plague many alcoholics in withdrawal. The law also gets rid of higher deductibles, higher cost-sharing, and limits on maximum payable amounts that aren't also included in a policy's medical coverage (in other words, the deductibles and so forth must be equal for mental health and medical and surgical conditions).

Covering the Uninsured

People who needed help to quit drinking in Dr. Jellinek's time may have benefited from a more compassionate view of their condition from doctors and the public, but treatment options were sparse compared to today's many options. That's one way problem drinkers had few choices. As treatment options multiplied over the ensuing decades, another problem emerged, which was a lack of insurance parity, a problem that was seemingly addressed with legislation like the MHPAEA. However, there still remains a large population of alcoholics and addicts with no access to treatment: the uninsured.

There is a huge financial cost for society to bear when it comes to covering the expenses related to people addicted to alcohol who don't have insurance. With no financial safety net, uninsured addicts are far less likely to receive treatment in the early, more treatable phase of their disorder. They are, therefore, more likely to wind up in an emergency room, where their chances for successful treatment are small. The expense of such visits generally reverts back to the hospital, which in turn must pass the cost along to its other consumers. Another scenario is that the drinker, with no resources for getting sober and successfully participating in work and family life, ends up on the street where he or she is likely to represent a public-health expense, either because of incarceration or publicly funded treatment programs. Ultimately, everyone pays the price for uninsured alcoholics.

More importantly, there is the human cost—having no access to healthcare merely compounds the misery of alcoholics, their loved ones, and members of the public who must contend with the fallout of addiction: increased crime and homelessness, broken families, a foster system full of children from unstable, alcohol-affected families, and more.

There is no easy answer to the problem of helping every person get insured. In the United States, proposed solutions include federally funded universal healthcare or increased public funding for people with substance-abuse disorders and no insurance. With millions of alcoholics still in need of treatment, such solutions are desperately needed to make sure that any person trying to stop drinking has the option to get help.

CONCLUSION

More and more, scientists and healthcare professionals are gaining a clearer understanding of alcoholism and addiction in general. Advanced clinical research, innovative therapies, and improved public awareness and support continue to emerge to give alcoholics greater odds of getting and staying sober. Considering how difficult it is for an alcoholic to resist the craving to drink, the more tools a doctor, a therapist, a family member, or a friend has to help a drinker combat addiction, the more likely it is that alcoholics everywhere will have the chance to lead fuller, healthier lives—and so will those around them. Although it has taken centuries for society to recognize, accept, and begin to understand alcoholism, experts today agree that treatment works.

Timeline

3000 BC–500 BC	Cultures throughout the Ancient World revere the mythical power of wine and worship various gods of wine, such as Dionysus (Greek), Osiris (Egyptian), and Bacchus (Roman).
1800 BC	The Babylonian King Hammurabi establishes a code of laws that regulate the sale and price of alcohol in taverns.
1100 AD	Distillation is first documented at a medical school in Salerno, Italy.
15th–16th centuries	Alcohol is used as a pain medication and anesthetic in hospitals throughout the western world. Distillation becomes common practice in Europe and alcohol abuse begins to be recognized as a social problem.
1606	The English Parliament passes the "Act to Repress the Odious and Loathsome Sin of Drunkenness."
1619	Public drunkenness is declared illegal in the colony of Virginia. Drunkenness is viewed as a sin and public drunkenness is punishable by a fine and a jail sentence.
1710–1750	Low grain prices and negative trade deficit cause an increase in England's production of gin known as the "English Gin

	Epidemic." The epidemic brings a sudden increase in infant mortality and birth defects.
1751	Parliament raises liquor taxes in order to curb the "English Gin Epidemic."
1777	Dr. Benjamin Rush, Surgeon General of the Colonial Army, launches a health education campaign to warn the public about alcohol-related health problems.
1779	During the Revolutionary War, the U.S.S. *Constitution* sets sail with 48,600 gallons of water and 74,400 gallons of rum listed on its manifest.
1804	Scottish physician Thomas Trotter writes *On Drunkenness and Its Effects on the Human Body*. Trotter is one of the first to view excessive drinking as a possible disease.
1851	The first American prohibition law is passed, prohibiting the sale of alcohol in Maine. Many other U.S. states follow Maine's lead and ban alcohol before the federal government passes the 18th Amendment.
1869	The National Prohibition Party is formed in the United States.
1870	Employers are no longer allowed to legally serve alcohol to workers on the job.
1874	The Woman's Christian Temperance Union is formed.
1906	The U.S. federal government passes the "Pure Food and Drug Act," which calls for the labeling of foods and beverages containing drugs, namely alcohol and cocaine.
1919	The 18th Amendment to the U.S. Constitution is ratified, effectively making America a "dry" country. The Amendment bans the manufacturing, distribution and sale of alcohol, but not the consumption of alcohol.
1929	The Great Depression contributes to the overturning of Prohibition due to the increased need for potential alcohol tax revenues and the significant number of jobs the alcohol industry is able to provide.
1935	Alcoholics Anonymous is formed.

1950s	The National Institutes of Health conduct the first in-depth investigations on the causes and effects of excessive alcohol consumption.
1956	The American Medical Association officially declares alcoholism a disease.
1969	Congress holds official hearings on alcoholism.
1970	The National Institute on Alcohol Abuse and Alcoholism is formed.
1970s	The legal drinking age in America is lowered from 21 to 18 years of age in most U.S. states.
1973	Fetal alcohol syndrome is officially documented.
1977	The first public warnings about fetal alcohol syndrome are administered.
1980s	Mothers Against Drunk Driving and Students Against Drunk Driving are formed and succeed in their lobbying efforts to return the legal drinking age to 21 years of age.
1989	Warning labels indicating that drinking alcohol can have adverse effects on the human body are required on all alcohol containers.
2001	Congress passes the Department of Transportation Appropriations Act of 2001, which establishes .08 as the national legal level for blood alcohol content while driving.
2007	Medical studies suggest that moderate consumption of alcohol is linked to increased risk of breast, rectal, and liver cancer in women and prostate cancer in men.
2008	Congress passes the Mental Health Parity and Addiction Equity Act of 2008.

Glossary

Abstinence: The state of being without a drug, such as alcohol, on which one is dependent.

Addiction: The continuous, compulsive use of a substance or participation in a specific act despite physical and psychological harm to the user and others.

Alcohol abuse: The act of engaging in excessive drinking that causes health or social problems without being dependent on alcohol or having fully lost control over its use.

Alcohol by volume (ABV): A worldwide standard measure of how much alcohol is contained in an alcoholic beverage.

Alcohol dependence: A physical dependence on alcohol.

Alcohol flush: Redness in the face after consuming a small amount of alcohol, caused by a deficiency in an enzyme that helps metabolize alcohol (ALDH2).

Alcohol poisoning: A dangerous and possibly deadly consequence of drinking large amounts of alcohol in a short period of time.

Alcoholic amnesia: Memory loss due to alcohol intoxication, possibly lasting from a few hours to several days.

Alcoholic cardiomyopathy: Heart muscle damage caused by excessive alcohol consumption, possibly leading to heart failure.

Alcoholic hepatitis: An inflammation of the liver caused by excessive alcohol use.

Alcoholic proof: A measure of how much alcohol is contained in an alcoholic beverage. Commonly used in the United States, it is defined as twice the percentage of alcohol by volume (ABV).

Alcoholism: A chronic disease characterized by the inability to control the consumption of alcoholic beverages.

Al kohl: An Arabic word, from which the word "alcohol" originates, that refers to fermented grains, fruits, or sugars that form an intoxicating beverage.

Binge drinking: The consumption of dangerously large quantities of alcoholic beverages in one session.

Biological: Of or pertaining to life and living things.

Blacking out: A period of alcoholic amnesia caused by intoxication, during which a person is physically active but mentally unable to form new memories or recall events once sober.

Blood alcohol content (BAC) or blood alcohol level (BAL): The concentration of alcohol in a person's blood, commonly used to measure intoxication for legal or medical purposes.

Bootlegging: The act of producing, distributing, or selling alcoholic liquors illegally, derived from a smuggler's practice of carrying liquor in the leg of one's boot.

Chronic illness: A disease that has a prolonged course, does not resolve spontaneously, and is rarely completely cured.

Cirrhosis: Irreversible scarring of the liver caused by liver damage from a chronic progressive condition such as long-term alcohol abuse.

Cognitive behavioral therapy (CBT): A form of psychotherapy based on the idea that a person's thoughts—not external effects such as people, situations, or events—cause his or her feelings and behaviors.

Compulsion: A strong, usually irresistible impulse to perform an act, especially one that is irrational or contrary to one's will.

Delirium tremens (DTs): A severe form of withdrawal that involves sudden and severe mental or neurological changes, such as body tremors, confusion, disorientation, delirium, and hallucinations.

Detoxification ("detox"): The process of removing a poison, toxin, or intoxicating or addictive substance from the body.

Distillation: The purification or concentration of a substance, obtaining the essence or volatile properties contained within it.

Environmental forces: The social and cultural factors that shape the life of a person or a population.

Fermentation: A change brought about by yeast enzymes converting grape sugar into ethyl alcohol.

Fetal alcohol effects (FAE): A pattern of negative physical, developmental, and psychological effects seen in babies born to mothers who drank alcohol during pregnancy.

Fetal alcohol syndrome (FAS): A disorder of permanent birth defects in children of women who consumed alcohol during pregnancy.

Genetics: How the characteristics of living things are transmitted from one generation to the next.

Hallucination: Perception of objects, sounds, or sensations having no reality, usually arising from a disorder of the nervous system, in response to certain drugs, or as a symptom of withdrawal from an addictive substance.

Inhibition: The conscious or unconscious suppression of free or spontaneous thought or behavior, such as enabling the delay of gratification from pleasurable activities.

Intoxication: When the quantity of alcohol a person consumes exceeds the individual's tolerance for alcohol, causing the person's mental and physical abilities to become impaired.

Liquor: A distilled or spirituous beverage, such as brandy or whiskey, as distinguished from a fermented beverage, such as wine or beer.

Liver: A large, reddish-brown organ located in the upper right portion of the abdominal cavity responsible for ridding the body of toxic substances.

Maintenance: The stage in which a person's sobriety is sustained for an extended period of time and part of everyday life.

Metabolism: The processing of a specific substance within the living body.

Neurological: Of or pertaining to the nervous system.

Passing out: Falling asleep or becoming unconscious from drinking excessive amounts of alcohol.

Prohibition: Legal prevention of manufacturing, transporting, and selling alcoholic beverages.

Psychological: Of or pertaining to the will or the mind and its function.

Rehabilitation ("rehab"): The process of physically restoring a sick or disabled person by therapeutic measures and education to enable participation in the activities of a normal life within the limitations of the person's physical disability.

Social: Of or pertaining to the life, welfare, and relations of human beings in a community.

Spirits: Unsweetened, distilled alcoholic beverages that have an alcohol content of at least 20 percent alcohol by volume (ABV).

Temperance: Moderation in or abstinence from the indulgence of a natural appetite or passion for alcoholic liquors.

Tolerance: Physiological resistance to a toxin.

Wernicke-Korsakoff syndrome: Thiamin (vitamin B-1) deficiency due to long-term alcohol use, possibly leading to brain damage.

Willpower: The control of one's impulses and actions.

Withdrawal (abstinence syndrome): Characteristic signs and symptoms that appear when a drug that causes physical or psychological dependence after extreme or extended use is suddenly discontinued or decreased.

Bibliography

Ackerman R. 1987. *Children of Alcoholics*. Simon & Schuster: New York.

Ackerman R. 1993. *Silent Sons*. Simon & Schuster: New York.

Aiseiri Research. *Courage to Change*.

Al-Anon Family Groups. 2006. Membership Survey: Survey among Alateen Members, Fall 2006. Available at: http://www.alanon.alateen.org/pdf/AlateenProfessionals.pdf.

Al-Anon Family Groups. 2006. Member Survey Results: Al-Anon Family Groups, Fall 2006. Available at: http://www.alanon.alateen.org/pdf/AlAnonProfessionals.pdf.

Alcoholics Anonymous. August 2008. Fact File. Available at: http://www.aa.org/pdf/products/m-24_aafactfile.pdf.

Alterman RL. 2008. "A Look to the Future of Alcoholism Treatment." LaChance Publishing.

American Council on Alcoholism. 2009. "Beyond 12 Steps." Available at: http://www.aca-usa.org/beyond12Steps.htm.

American Psychiatric Association. 2000. "Diagnostic and Statistical Manual of Mental Disorders DSM-IV-TR." 4th ed. Washington D.C.: American Psychiatric Publishing.

Anti-Saloon League. July 2008. Available at: http://www.wpl.lib.oh.us/AntiSaloon/history/history.html.

Barr A. 1999. *Drink: A Social History of America*. New York: Carroll & Graf Publishers.

Bayard M, et al. 2004. "Alcohol Withdrawal Syndrome." American Family Physician.

Behr E. 1996. *Prohibition: Thirteen Years that Changed America*. New York: Arcade Publishing.

Berk L. 2004. "Temperance and Prohibition Era Propaganda: A Study in Rhetoric." Alcohol, Temperance, & Prohibition. Available at: http://dl.lib.brown.edu/temperance/essay.html.

Berry M. September 2007. "Employers Blame Alcohol for Employee Absence and Lost Productivity." Available at: http://www.personneltoday.com/articles/2007/09/17/42374/employers-blame-alcohol-for-employee-absence-and-lost-productivity.html.

Beyer R. 2003. *The Greatest Stories Never Told*. New York: HarperCollins.

Blume S. 2000. "Treatment of Substance Misuse in the New Century." *West J Med* 172(1): 4–5.

Boston University School of Public Health. May 2003. "Study Links Early Alcohol Use and Behavior Problems in Young Adulthood." Available at: http://www.jointogether.org/news/research/pressreleases/2003/study-links-early-alcohol-use.html.

Briggs J. 2005. *Lincoln's Speeches Reconsidered*. Baltimore: Johns Hopkins University Press.

Brown University. 2008. "Alcoholism and Your Body." Available at: http://www.brown.edu/Student_Services/Health_Services/Health_Education/atod/alc_aayb.htm.

Bureau of Justice Statistics. April 1998. "Alcohol and Crime." Available at: http://www.ojp.usdoj.gov/bjs/pub/pdf/ac.pdf.

Burge SK, and Schneider FD. January 1999. "Alcohol-Related Problems: Recognition and Intervention." *American Family Physician*.

Caces M, et al. Summer 1991. "Alcohol Use and Physically Risky Behavior among Adolescents." *Alcohol Health & Research World*.

California Department of Alcohol and Drug Programs. 2002. Driving Under-the-Influence (DUI) Statistics. Driving Under-the-Influence Branch. Available at: www.adp.ca.gov.

Centers for Disease Control and Prevention. 2008. "Impaired Driving." Available at: http://www.cdc.gov/ncipc/factsheets/drving.htm.

Centers for Disease Control and Prevention. 2009. "Motor Vehicle Safety." Available at: http://www.cdc.gov/Motorvehiclesafety/index.html.

Centers for Disease Control and Prevention. 2008. "Quick Stats on Underage Drinking." Available at: http://www.cdc.gov/Alcohol/quickstats/underage_drinking.htm.

Chen CM, and Yi H. 2007. "Trends in Alcohol-Related Morbidity Among Short-Stay Community Hospital Discharges, United States, 1979–2005." Bethesda, MD: National Institutes of Health, National Institute on Alcohol Abuse and Alcoholism. Surveillance Report #80. Available at: http://pubs.niaaa.nih.gov/publications/surveillance80/HDS05.pdf.

Clarke J. 2006. "LSD Helps Alcoholics Put Down the Bottle."*Independent News*.

Cleveland Clinic. February 2007. "FAQs on Alcohol and Alcoholism." Available at: http://my.clevelandclinic.org/disorders/alcoholism/hic_FAQs_on_Alcohol_Abuse_and_Alcoholism.aspx.

Columbia University. 2009. "Alcohol & Sexual Assault." Available at: http://www.health.columbia.edu/docs/topics/sexual_violence/alcohol_assault.html.

Conrad P. 1980. *Deviance and Medicalization: From Badness to Sickness*. New York: Mosby.

Crews E. 2007. "Rattle-Skull, Stonewall, Bogus, Blackstrap, Bombo, Mimbo, Whistle Belly, Syllabub, Sling, Toddy, and Flip: Drinking in Colonial America." *Journal of Colonial Williamsburg Foundation*. Available at: http://www.history.org/Foundation/journal/Holiday07/drink.cfm.

Dawson DA, Grant BF, and Li TK. 2005. "Quantifying the Risks Associated with Exceeding Recommended Drinking Limits." Alcoholism Clinical and Experimental Research. 29: 902–908. Available at: http://www.ncbi.nlm.nih.gov/pubmed/15897737.

Dee T. 2001. "Alcohol Abuse and Economic Conditions: Evidence from Repeated Cross-Sections of Individual-Level Data." *Health Economics* 10(3): 257–270.

Denyssen J. June 1956. "Medical Hypnosis." *S.A. Journal of Medicine*.

Dillon P. 2003. *The Much Lamented Death of Madam Geneva: The Eighteenth Century Gin Craze*. Boston: Justin, Charles & Co., Publishers.

Donovan M, et al. July 2005. "Quality of Life as an Outcome Measure in Alcoholism Treatment Research." *Journal of Studies on Alcohol*.

Douglass F. 1845. 1845–1846. "Intemperance and Slavery: An Address Delivered in Cork, Ireland, on October 20, 1845," *Truth Seeker*, 1: 142–144.

Drucker E. 1998. "Drug Prohibition and Public Health." Public Health Reports. U.S. Public Health Service. Vol. 114.

Dunlap M. 2006. Social History of Alcohol Use and Abuse. Available at: http://www.michaeledunlap.com/#id_11700126094151686.

Dyck E. 2006. "Hitting Highs at Rock Bottom: LSD Treatment for Alcoholism, 1950–1970." *Social History of Medicine*. Available at: http://shm.oxfordjournals.org/cgi/content/abstract/19/2/313.

EMQ Children & Family Services. 2007. "Facts about Drug and Alcohol Abuse." Available at: http://www.emq.org/press/faq/addiction.html.

Engs RC, Diebold BA, and Hansen DJ. 1996. "The Drinking Patterns and Problems of a National Sample of College Students, 1994." *Journal of Alcohol and Drug Education* 41(3): 13–33.

Enoch MA, and Goldman D. February 1, 2002. "Problem Drinking and Alcoholism: Diagnosis and Treatment." *American Family Physician*.

European Commission. 2008. "Alcohol Abuse Blighting Lives Across the EU." Available at: http://ec.europa.eu/news/environment/080416_1_en.htm.

Farley B. "The Evolution of Chemical Dependency Treatment and Services in Washington State: Historical Time Line 1800's–1930's." Available at: file:///c:/Users/Rich/Desktop/Alcoho20Book/timeline_washington_state.html.

Fuller R, and Hiller-Sturmhöfel S. 1999. "Alcoholism Treatment in the United States: An Overview." *Alcohol Research & Health* 23(2).

Garrett F. 2002. "Your First AA Meeting: An Unofficial Guide For the Perplexed." Psychiatry and Wellness: Behavioral Medicine Associates, Atlanta and Alpharetta. Available at: http://www.bmawellness.com/papers/First_AA_Meeting.html.

George Washington University Medical Center. 2009. "State Laws, Health Insurance, and Alcohol Treatment." Available at: http://www.ensuringsolutions.org/resources/resources_show.htm?doc_id=332865.

Getz O. 1978. *Whiskey: An American Pictorial History*. New York: Dave McKay Company.

Goodwin D, Gebrielli W, Penick E, Nickel E, Chhibber S, Knop J, Jensen P, and Schulsinger F. 1999. "Breast-Feeding and Alcoholism: The Trotter Hypothesis." *American Journal of Psychiatry*.

Hanson D. 2007. "Puritans to Prohibition." Alcohol Problems and Solutions. Available at: http://www2.potsdam.edu/hansondj/funfacts/PuritansToProhibition.html.

Hazelden Foundation. 1993. *The Twelve Steps of Alcoholics Anonymous*. Minnesota: Hazelden Foundation.

Henningfield JE. 1994. National Institute on Drug Abuse. "Addictive Properties of Popular Drugs." Available at: http://drugwarfacts.org/cms/?q=node/28.

Hermann R, Dorwart R, Hoover C, and Brody J. 1995. "Variation in ECT Use in the United States." *American Journal of Psychiatry* 152(6): 869–875.

Herrick and Herrick. 2007. *100 Questions and Answers about Alcoholism*. Massachusetts: Jones and Bartlett Publishers.

Hingson R, Heeren T, and Winter M. 1996. "Lowering State Legal Blood Alcohol Limits to 0.08%: The Effect on Fatal Motor Vehicle Crashes." *Public Health Brief* 86(9): 1297–1299.

Hingson R, Heeren T, and Winter M. 1994. "Lower Legal Blood Alcohol Limits for Young Drivers." *Public Health Reports* 109: 738–744.

Hingson R, Heeren T, and Winter M. 1999. "Preventing Impaired Driving." *Alcohol Research & Health* 23(1).

Hingson R, Heeren T, Zakocs R, Kopstein A, and Wechsler H. 2005. "Magnitude of Alcohol-Related Mortality and Morbidity Among U.S. College Students Ages 18–24: Changes from 1998 to 2001." *Annual Review of Public Health* 26: 259–279.

Housecroft CE, and Sharpe AG. 2001. *Inorganic Chemistry* (2nd edition). New York: Pearson/Prentice Hall.

Howard J. 2006. "Alcoholism: The Family Disease." Available at: www.mobar.org/8167bdac -a222-4d09-b83f-5c4f90d3e1bf.aspx.

Institute of Alcohol Studies. January 2009. "Adolescents and Alcohol." Institute of Alcohol Studies.

Institute for Health Policy. 2001. "Substance Abuse: The Nation's Number One Health Problem." Brandeis University.

Insurance Institute for Highway Safety. 2009. DUI/DWI Laws. Available at: http://www.iihs.org/laws/dui.aspx.

Jarjour S, et al. 2009. "Effect of Acute Ethanol Administration on the Release of Opioid Peptides from the Midbrain Including the Ventral Tegmental Area." *Alcoholism: Clinical and Experimental Research*.

Jellinek EM. 1972. *The Disease Concept of Alcoholism*. New Haven, CT: College and University Press.

Johnson BA, et al. 2007. "Topiramate for Treating Alcohol Dependence." *Journal of the American Medical Association* 298: 1641–1651. Available at: http://jama.ama-assn.org/cgi/content/full/298/14/1641.

Kaiser Family Foundation. September 2008. "Sexual Health of Adolescents in the United States." Kaiser Family Foundation.

Kershaw and Guidot. 2008. "Alcoholic Lung Disease." *Alcohol Research and Health* 38(1).

Ketcham K, and Asbury W. 2000. *Beyond the Influence: Understanding and Defeating Alcoholism*. New York: Bantam Books.

Kinney J. 2009. *Loosening the Grip: A Handbook of Alcohol Information*. New York: McGraw-Hill.

Kittleson MJ, and Youngerman B. 2005. *The Truth about Alcohol*. New York: Facts on File.

Kobler J. 1993. *Ardent Spirits: The Rise and Fall of Prohibition*. Da Capo Press.

Kyriacou DN, et al. December 1999. "Risk Factors for Injury to Women from Domestic Violence." *New England Journal of Medicine* 25(341): 1892–1898.

Lapham S. 2004. "Screening and Brief Intervention in the Criminal Justice System." *Alcohol Research & Health*.

Lee H. 1963. *How Dry We Were: Prohibition Revisited*, EngleWood Cliffs: Prentice Hall Inc.

Leshner A. June 2001. "What Does It Mean That Addiction Is a Brain Disease?" *Monitor on Psychology* 32(5).

Levinson D. 2002. *The Encyclopedia of Crime and Punishment.* Thousand Oaks, CA: Sage Publications.

Lincoln A. 1843. "Temperance Address: An Address Delivered before the Springfield (Illinois) Washington Temperance Society, on the 22d February, 1842." *Sangamo Journal* March 25, 1842.

Lovinger DM. 1997. "Serotonin's Role in Alcohol's Effects on the Brain." *Alcohol Health & Research World* 21(2).

Marin Institute. 2006. "Alcohol and Violence." Available at: http://www.marininstitute .org/alcohol_policy/violence.htm.

Mayo Clinic. May 2008. "Alcoholism." Available at: http://www.mayoclinic.com/ health/alcoholism/DS00340.

McCaig LF, and Burt CW. 2005. "National Hospital Ambulatory Medical Care Survey: 2003 Emergency Department Summary." Advance Data from Vital and Health Statistics; No. 358. Hyattsville, Maryland: National Center for Health Statistics. Available at: http://www.cdc.gov/nchs/data/ad/ad358.pdf.

Medical News Today. September 2006. "Binge-drinking Teenagers At Greater Risk of Becoming Victims of Violence." Available at: http://www.medicalnewstoday .com/articles/52845.php.

Medline Plus. February 2008. "Alcoholism." Available at: http://www.nlm.nih.gov/ medlineplus/ency/article/000944.htm.

Mikalson J. 2005. *Ancient Greek Religion.* Malden, MA: Blackwell Publishing.

Miller J. 2007. "Alcoholism: Vice or Disease? A Conversation with Howard Fields." University of California, San Francisco. Available at: http://www.ucsf.edu/science-cafe/conversations/fields/.

Mintzer R. 2005. *Alcohol=Busted.* Berkeley Heights, NJ: Enslow Publishers.

Mokdad AH, Marks JS, Stroup DF, and Gerberding JL. 2004. "Actual Causes of Death in the United States, 2000." *Journal of the American Medical Association* 291(10): 1238–1245. Available at: http://www.ncbi.nlm.nih.gov/pubmed/15010446.

Morse RM, and Flavin DK. 1992. "The Definition of Alcoholism. The Joint Committee of the National Council on Alcoholism and Drug Dependence and the American Society of Addiction Medicine to Study the Definition and Criteria for the Diagnosis of Alcoholism." *Journal of the American Medical Association* 268(8): 1012–1014.

Mukamal KJ, et al. January 9, 2003. "Roles of Drinking Pattern and Type of Alcohol Consumed in Coronary Heart Disease in Men." *New England Journal of Medicine* 348(2): 109–118.

National Highway Safety Administration. August 2008. "2007 Traffic Safety Annual Assessment—Alcohol-Impaired Driving Fatalities." National Highway Safety Administration.

National Institute on Alcohol Abuse and Alcoholism. January 1995. "Alcohol-Medication Interactions." Alcohol Alert, No. 27.

National Institute on Alcohol Abuse and Alcoholism. December 1999. "Are Women More Vulnerable to Alcohol's Effects?" Alcohol Alert, No. 46.

National Institute on Alcohol Abuse and Alcoholism. October 1995. "Diagnostic Criteria for Alcohol Abuse and Dependence." Alcohol Alert, No. 30.

National Institute on Alcohol Abuse and Alcoholism. February 2007. "FAQs for the General Public." Available at: http://www.niaaa.nih.gov/FAQs/General-English/default.htm.

National Institute on Alcohol Abuse and Alcoholism. December 2000. "Fetal Alcohol Exposure and the Brain." Alcohol Alert, No. 50.

National Institute on Alcohol Abuse and Alcoholism. July 2003. "The Genetics of Alcoholism." Alcohol Alert, No. 60.

National Institute on Alcohol Abuse and Alcoholism. April 1992. "Moderate Drinking." Alcohol Alert, No. 16.

National Institute on Alcohol Abuse and Alcoholism. October 2000. "New Advances in Alcoholism Treatment." Alcohol Alert, No. 49.

National Institute on Alcohol Abuse and Alcoholism. July 1997. "Youth Drinking: Risk Factors and Consequences." Alcohol Alert, No. 37.

National Institute on Alcohol Abuse and Alcoholism. July 2004. "Alcohol: An Important Women's Health Issue." Alcohol Alert, No. 62.

National Institute on Alcohol Abuse and Alcoholism. April 1991. "Assessing Alcoholism." Alcohol Alert, No. 12.

National Institutes of Health. 2008. MedlinePlus. "Disulfiram." Available at: http://www.nlm.nih.gov/medlineplus/druginfo/meds/a682602.html.

Nemours Foundation. August 2006. "What Is Binge Drinking?" Available at: http://kidshealth.org/teen/drug_alcohol/alcohol/binge_drink.html.

Overstreet DH, et al. 2008. "Electroacupuncture Reduces Voluntary Alcohol Intake in Alcohol-Preferring Rats Via an Opiate-Sensitive Mechanism." Neurochemical Research 33(10): 2166–2170.

Parsons T. 2003. "Alcoholism and Its Effects on the Family." Allpsych Journal. Available at: www.allpysch.com/journal.

Pennsylvania Health System. "Historical Timeline: Dr. Benjamin Rush." Available at: www.uphs.upenn.edu/paharc/timeline.

Rea F. 1956. Alcoholism, Its Psychology and Cure. London: Epworth Press.

Reuters Health Information. October 2007. "Deep Brain Stimulation May Overcome Alcohol Dependence, Case Suggests." Available at: http://medgenmed.medscape.com/viewarticle/564797.

Rollnick S, and Miller WR. 1995. "What Is MI?" Available at: http://motivationalinterview.org/clinical/whatismi.html.

Rorabaugh R. 1979. The Alcoholic Republic: An American Tradition. New York: Oxford University Press.

Rotskoff L. 2002. Love on the Rocks: Men, Women and Alcohol in Post-World War II America. Chapel Hill: University of North Caroline Press.

Ruark J. 2000. "Interview: Addiction Is a Choice with Jeffery Schaler." Chronicle of Higher Education. Available at: http://www.schaler.net/addictionisachoice/interview.html.

Rutledge PC, Park A, and Sher KJ. 2008. "21st Birthday Drinking: Extremely Extreme." Journal of Consulting and Clinical Psychology 76(3): 511–516. Available at: http://www.apa.org/journals/releases/ccp763511.pdf.

Schaler J. 2000. Addiction Is a Choice. Chicago: Open Court Publishers.

Science Daily. April 2008. "Why People Engage in Risky Behavior While Intoxicated: Imaging Study Provides Glimpse of Alcohol's Effect On Brain." Available at: http://www.sciencedaily.com/releases/2008/04/080429204252.htm.

Scottish Parliament. 2008. *Costs of Alcohol Use and Misuse in Scotland.* Crown Copyright. Available at: http://www.scotland.gov.uk/Publications/2008/05/06091510/0.

Silverstein H. 1990. *Alcoholism.* New York: Franklin Watts.

SMART Recovery. 2009. Available at: http://smartrecovery.org.

Sourina J-C. 1990. *A History of Alcoholism.* Oxford: Basil Blackwell.

Stug DL, Priyadarsini S, and Hyman MM. 1986. "Alcohol Interventions: Historical and Sociocultural Approaches."

Substance Abuse and Mental Health Services Administration. "Who's Using Alcohol." Available at: http://family.samhsa.gov/talk/alcohol.aspx.

Thun MJ, et al. December 1997. "Alcohol Consumption and Mortality among Middle-Aged and Elderly U.S. Adults." *New England Journal of Medicine* 337: 1705–1714.

Trotter T. 1989 (facsimile of 1804 edition). "An Essay, Medical, Philosophical, and Chemical, on Drunkenness and its Effects on the Human Body". London: Routledge.

University of Rochester. August 2008. "Alcohol Use, Abuse and Dependency." Available at: http://www.rochester.edu/uhs/healthtopics/Alcohol/abuse.html.

U.S. Department of Health and Human Services. August 2005. "A Family History of Alcoholism. Are You at Risk?" NIH Publication No. 03-5340.

U.S. Department of Health and Human Services. January 2005. "Alcohol: A Women's Health Issue." NIH Publication No. 04–4956.

U.S. Department of Health and Human Services. 2005. "Dietary Guidelines for Americans." Available at: http://www.cnpp.usda.gov/Publications/DietaryGuidelines/2005/2005DGPolicyDocument.pdf.

U.S. Department of Health and Human Services 2008. "Impaired Driving Fact Sheet." Centers for Disease Control and Prevention.

U.S. Department of Health and Human Services. 2008. "The NSDUH Report: State Estimates of Persons Aged 18 or Older Driving Under the Influence of Alcohol or Illicit Drugs." Substance Abuse and Mental Health Services Administration Office of Applied Studies. Rockville, MD.

U.S. Department of Health and Human Services. 2008. "The NSDUH Report: Underage Alcohol Use: Where Do Young People Drink?" Substance Abuse and Mental Health Services Administration, Office of Applied Studies. Rockville, MD.

U.S. Department of Health and Human Services. 2008. "Americans Believe in Prevention and Recovery from Addictions." Substance Abuse and Mental Health Services Administration, Office of Applied Studies. Rockville, MD.

U.S. Department of Health and Human Services. 2008. "National Survey on Drug Use & Health." Substance Abuse and Mental Health Services Administration Office of Applied Studies. Rockville, MD.

U.S. Department of Health and Human Services. 2008. "Alcohol-Related Disease Impact." Centers for Disease Control and Prevention. Available at: http://www.cdc.gov/alcohol/ardi.htm.

U.S. Department of Health and Human Services. 2007. "What Colleges Need to Know Now: An Update on College Drinking Research." National Institutes of Health, National Institute of Alcohol Abuse and Alcoholism, National Advisory Council on Alcohol Abuse and Alcoholism, Task Force on College Drinking.

U.S. Department of Health and Human Services. 2007. "College Drinking Changing the Culture: A Snapshot of Drinking Consequences." National Institutes of Health,

National Institute of Alcohol Abuse and Alcoholism. Available at: www.collegedrinkingprevention.gov.

U.S. Department of Health and Human Services. 2004. "Largest Ever Comorbidity Study Reports Prevalence and Co-Occurrence of Alcohol, Drug, Mood and Anxiety Disorders." National Institutes of Health. Available at: www.nih.gov.

U.S. Department of Health and Human Services. 2002. "High-Risk Drinking in College: What We Know and What We Need to Learn." National Institute of Health, National Institute of Alcohol Abuse and Alcoholism, National Advisory Council on Alcohol Abuse and Alcoholism, Task Force on College Drinking.

U.S. Department of Health and Human Services. 2000. "Updating Estimates of the Economic Costs of Alcohol Abuse in the United States: Estimates, Update Methods and Data." Public Health Service, National Institutes of Health and National Institute of Alcohol Abuse and Alcoholism. Available at: www.niaaa.nih.gov.

U.S. Department of Labor. 2008. "Fact Sheet: The Mental Health Parity Act." Available at: http://www.dol.gov/ebsa/newsroom/fsmhparity.html.

U.S. Department of Treasury. 2008. "Budget-in-Brief." Office of Performance Budgeting and Strategic Planning.

U.S. Food and Drug Administration. May 1996. "Medications Can Aid Recovery from Alcoholism." Available at: http://www.fda.gov/FDAC/features/496_alco.html.

Valenzuela CF. 1997. "Alcohol and Neurotransmitter Interactions." *Alcohol Health & Research World* 21(2).

Vassoler FM, et al. August 2008. "Deep Brain Stimulation of the Nucleus Accumbens Shell Attenuates Cocaine Priming-Induced Reinstatement of Drug Seeking in Rats." *Journal of Neuroscience* 28(35): 8735–8739.

Virginia Tech. 2009. "Factors that Affect Intoxication." Available at: http://www.alcohol.vt.edu/Students/alcoholEffects/intoxFactors.htm.

Washton A. 1990. "Structured Outpatient Treatments of Alcohol vs. Drug Dependencies." In *Recent Developments in Alcoholism*, Vol 8. Ed. Marc Galanter. New York: Plenum Press.

White W. 1998. *Slaying the Dragon: The History of Addiction in America.* Bloomington, IL: Chestnut Health Systems.

Youngerman B. 2005. *The Truth about Alcohol.* Kittleson M, ed. New York: Book Builders.

Index

Polk State College
Lakeland Library

About the Author

MARIA GIFFORD is an independent health writer in Rochester, Minnesota. She has produced evidence-based consumer health content for the Mayo Clinic, the American Diabetes Association, Time Inc., Rodale, and *Ladies' Home Journal*.

About the Advisor

BRUCE PHARISS, M.D., is a board-certified psychiatrist and diplomate of the American Board of Psychiatry and Neurology in addiction psychiatry. He is a clinical assistant professor of psychiatry at Weill Medical College of Cornell University in New York City, where he lectures on diagnosis and treatment of substance abuse disorders. Dr. Phariss maintains private practices in Manhattan, New York, and Montclair, New Jersey, specializing in addiction psychiatry, psychotherapy, and psychopharmacology.

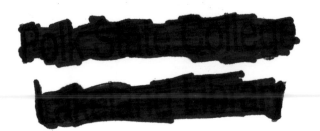